Cipro® TABLETS

MILES

MILES

(ciprofloxacin HCl/Miles)

OUTPATIENT ANTIMICROBIAL THERAPY: RECENT ADVANCES

EDITED BY

George A. Pankey, M.D.

and

Geoffrey H. Kalish, M.D.

HEALTH CARE COMMUNICATIONS, INC. CLIFTON, NEW JERSEY

OUTPATIENT ANTIMICROBIAL THERAPY: RECENT ADVANCES

Library of Congress Catalog Card Number: 89-81071

ISBN: 0-945986-12-2

Cover design by Rita Rovazzi

Contents

Introduction

The appropriate use of antimicrobials in an outpatient setting has become critical for the busy practicing physician. Because of a general heightened awareness of the escalating cost of inpatient medical care and the recent development of new very potent antimicrobials, this book will hopefully provide the most up-to-date plan of action for the nonhospitalized patient requiring antimicrobial therapy. We believe the authors of the chapters in this book have accomplished this goal.

The first section of this book comprises two chapters devoted to general, but important topics. A brief history of the use of antimicrobials in an outpatient setting is provided by Lawrence J. Eron, M.D. in Chapter 1. Data now support the cost-effective outpatient treatment of a wide range of infections. In Chapter 2, Irwin H. Rosenstock, Ph.D. discusses aspects of the patient-physician relationship that relate to compliance with medical advice. Reasons for lack of patient compliance with a therapeutic regime are given, as well as methods for improvement.

The next three chapters focus on a group of related infections. In Chapter 3, H. Hunter Handsfield, M.D. discusses general principles and specifics for the treatment of common sexually transmitted diseases. Particular attention is given to treatment of the patient with multiple infections and to newer therapeutic agents. Providing a number of diagnostic pearls, in Chapter 4, Alan S. Berkeley, M.D. discusses the outpatient management of gynecologic infections, especially vaginitis and pelvic inflammatory disease. Relevant information is presented to allow the clinician to determine whether or not to treat a specific patient in an ambulatory or hospital setting. In Chapter 5, Joseph R. Dalovisio, M.D. discusses the many newer agents available for the outpatient therapy of urinary tract infections.

Two chapters deal with skin, skin structure and bone infections. In Chapter 6, George A. Pankey, M.D. provides the clinician with the latest thoughts on treatment of skin and skin structure infections, running the gamut from impetigo to skin infections associated with water contamination. Ambulatory therapy of osteomyelitis in a cost-conscious environment is presented by Layne O. Gentry, M.D. in Chapter 7. While intravenous therapy remains the standard, the early success of the fluoroquinolones and other potent new antimicrobials promises a much shorter hospitalization for patients with osteomyelitis.

The respiratory tract is the prime focus of the next two chapters. In Chapter 8, Jerome O. Klein, M.D. evaluates currently available therapies for use in the upper respiratory infections of children. Also discussed are other special considerations in the outpatient antibiotic treatment of children, e.g., meningitis prophylaxis. Traditional therapy and use of newer agents for the treatment of lower respiratory tract infections are discussed in Chapter 9, by Louis D. Saravolatz, M.D.

The remaining two chapters in the book discuss problems that are greatly benefitted by the advent of newer antimicrobials. In Chapter 10, Herbert L. DuPont, M.D. discusses the management of acute gastrointestinal infections, delineating those requiring antimicrobial therapy from those expected to resolve without such therapy. Finally, in Chapter 11, Laurence M. Cortez, M.D. provides an excellent discussion of some of the latest thinking on outpatient therapy for infections in patients with AIDS, dosing parenterally, orally or by inhalation.

Overall, there is a clear message: the availability of antimicrobial agents, highly effective with infrequent dosing, parenterally or orally, allows a greater number of infections to be treated on an outpatient basis, thereby decreasing the cost of medical care and minimizing disruption to the lives of patients and their families.

George A. Pankey, M.D.
Geoffrey H. Kalish, M.D.
September, 1989

Contributors

Alan S. Berkeley, M.D.
Chief of Gynecology
The New York Hospital
Associate Professor of Obstetrics and Gynecology
Cornell University Medical College
New York, New York

Laurence M. Cortez, M.D.
Associate Head, Section of Infectious Disease
Ochsner Clinic and Alton Ochsner Foundation
New Orleans, Louisiana

Joseph R. Dalovisio, M.D.
Staff Member, Section of Infectious Disease
Ochsner Clinic and Alton Ochsner Foundation
New Orleans, Louisiana

Herbert L. DuPont, M.D.
Professor of Medicine
Director of the Program in Infectious Diseases
University of Texas Medical School
Houston, Texas

Lawrence J. Eron, M.D., F.A.C.P.
Division of Infectious Disease
Fairfax Hospital
Clinical Associate Professor of Medicine
Georgetown University School of Medicine
Washington, D.C.

Layne O. Gentry, M.D.
Chief, Infectious Disease Section
St. Luke's Episcopal Hospital
Clinical Professor of Medicine, Microbiology and Immunology
Baylor College of Medicine
Houston, Texas

H. Hunter Handsfield, M.D.
Professor of Medicine
University of Washington School of Medicine
Director, Sexually Transmitted Disease Control Program
Seattle-King County Department of Public Health
Seattle, Washington

Geoffrey H. Kalish, M.D.
President and Medical Director
Health Care Communications, Inc.
Clifton, New Jersey

Jerome O. Klein, M.D.
Director, Division of Pediatric Infectious Disease
Boston City Hospital
Professor of Pediatrics
Boston University School of Medicine
Boston, Massachusetts

George A. Pankey, M.D.
Head, Section of Infectious Disease
Ochsner Clinic and Alton Ochsner Foundation
New Orleans, Louisiana

Irwin M. Rosenstock, Ph.D.
FHP Endowed Professor and Director
Center for Health Behavior Studies
California State University, Long Beach
Long Beach, California

Louis D. Saravolatz, M.D.
Clinical Professor of Medicine
University of Michigan
Division Head, Infectious Disease and Hospital Epidemiology
Henry Ford Hospital
Detroit, Michigan

CHAPTER 1

Outpatient Antimicrobial Therapy: A Brief History

Lawrence J. Eron, M.D., F.A.C.P.
Fairfax, Virginia

INTRODUCTION

Before the availability of general anesthesia and effective antimicrobials, confinement to a hospital was associated with an extremely high mortality rate and was to be avoided at all costs. Unfortunately, the impoverished required hospitalization because the home environment did not allow effective care. The well-heeled, on the other hand, were cared for as outpatients, usually by physicians and hired private nurses. Relatives accepted responsibility for the day-to-day care of the ill within their own family.

In 1796, the Boston Dispensary organized the first outpatient program in the United States to care for discharged inpatients using lay help and paraprofessionals. In 1877 the women's branch of the New York City Mission standardized their professional outpatient staff by employing graduate nurses to care for the sick at home. In 1885, a voluntary nursing agency was founded in Buffalo, and that agency ultimately became the Visiting Nurses Association (VNA).[1]

The practice of using graduate nurses to care for outpatients, started by the New York City Mission, was adopted in 1898 by the Los Angeles County Health Department, the first municipal health department to participate in home services. In 1909, the private sector became involved when the Metropolitan Life Insurance Company offered home health services. By 1928, the Metropolitan Life Insurance Company operated 953 facilities providing home health services.

THE HOSPITAL WITHOUT WALLS

In 1941, an outpatient program was established at Syracuse University, that better integrated the hospital and outpatient arenas. In 1947, Dr. E. M. Bluestone took the process one step further by developing what he called a "hospital without walls." This was conceived as a single program with similar staffing for both inpatients and outpatients. Unified medical records were kept for both, and a joint program was organized for nursing and medication orders, occupational and physical therapy, social services, housekeeping services, and patient transportation. Indeed, the medical service itself was not divided into outpatient and inpatient departments. The result of this unified approach was a smoother transition from inpatient to outpatient status.[1]

MEDICARE AND OUTPATIENT PROGRAMS

Similar programs "without walls" proliferated during the early 1950's. In 1958, the Surgeon General's National Advisory Commission on Chronic Disease and Health of the Aged organized a conference on home care in Roanoke, Virginia. This, the first attempt at standardization of the delivery of home services to patients, culminated in the passage of the Medicare Act in 1965. In order to be licensed and to receive remuneration, Medicare required home health care agencies to provide not only nursing services but also other types of therapy. This concept of "nursing service plus one," frequently linked outpatient nursing with occupational therapy, physical therapy, speech therapy, social services and the like. Notably, at the time of enactment of the 1965 Medicare Act, of 1,100 home health care agencies, only 250 were considered qualified for reimbursement under the new standards. With an immediate infusion of $16 million in government funds to upgrade home health care agencies in 1966, 1,275 were able to be certified under the new regulations.[1]

INTRAVENOUS ANTIBIOTIC THERAPY IN OUTPATIENT SETTINGS

At about the same time as the standardization of outpatient therapy by Medicare, new and extremely potent antibiotics were developed which required intravenous infusion. These new antibiotics (methicillin and gentamicin, respectively) were primarily for the treatment of infections caused by staphylococci that were penicillin-resistant and by gram-negative bacilli that were resistant to the oral antibiotics ampicillin, tetracycline, and chloramphenicol. In 1974, Rucker and Harrison reported on a series of 62 patients with cystic fibrosis treated by outpatient parenteral antibiotics.[2] This was the first published report demonstrating that patients with serious infections requiring parenteral antibiotics could be treated in an outpatient setting. In 1978, Antoniskis and colleagues compared 13 outpatients with seven inpatients, all of whom received intravenous antibiotic therapy.[3] The results of therapy were comparable, suggesting that outpatient therapy was a viable therapeutic option. Similarly encouraging results were obtained by Stiver's group[4] and by Kind and associates[5] confirming the earlier findings. In 1982, our group published results of a series of 150 patients treated by intravenous antibiotics in an outpatient setting[6] and the following year, Rehm and Weinstein described a series of 48 patients.[7] Both reports demonstrated that a wide variety of different infections could be treated in outpatients at a tremendous cost savings compared to inpatient therapy (Table I.).

TABLE I. Cost analysis (from reference 7)

Year	Average Hospital Cost*	Average Outpatient Cost**	Average Net Savings per Course	Average Daily Savings
	$	$	$	$
1979	2886	660	2226	212
1980	5409	1441	3968	235
1981	6100	1495	4605	276
1982	8991	1870	7121	339
Mean	7380	1652	5728	305

* *Includes daily room physician fees, antibiotic agents, and supplies.*

** *Includes daily physicians fees, antibiotic agents, laboratory studies, and supplies.*

A cost analysis comparing outpatient to inpatient therapy in four different types of hospitals confirmed these results (Table II.).[8]

TABLE II. Cost of care per patient with osteomyelitis treated (from reference 8)

Conventional vs Early Discharge

Inpatient	**Conventional Inpatient Treatment**			**Early Discharge Treatment**			
Data Source	**Direct Costs**	**Indirect Costs**	**Total Costs**	**Direct Costs**	**Indirect Costs**	**Total Costs**	**Savings**
NJDRG-MT*	$2,401	$380	$2,781	$1,971	$300	$2,271	$ 510
MDCRC-T**	5,583	380	5,943	3,524	300	3,824	2,119
Hospital A*	30,872	916	31,788	8,918	638	9,556	22,232
AAMC	4,536	402	4,938	3,023	319	3,342	1,596
Medicare DRG II	4,913	275	5,188	3,973	204	4,177	1,011

* *NJDRG-MT indicates the payment for patients with osteomyelitis in teaching hospitals in the New Jersey diagnosis related group (DRG) prospective payment system.*

** *MDCRC-T indicates the rate-regulated charges of Maryland teaching hospitals.*
* *Hospital A indicates the charges of a major urban teaching hospital.*

AAMC indicates the results of a survey of cost-to-charge ratios for different diagnostic groups at 24 member hospitals of the Association of American Medical Colleges.

Medicare DRG II represents the prospective payment rate for osteomyelitis established by the Health Care Financing Administration for Medicare's DRG prospective payment program.

Beginning in the late 1970's, many commercial agencies began offering home delivery of antimicrobial agents. Our group, Intracare, employed a rather unique ambulatory clinic model that differed from the home visit concept primarily because patients returned to us twice weekly for examination of their infection, for change of heparin locks, for more antibiotic resuspended in minibags, and for evaluation of adverse drug reactions. We found that two-thirds of our patients appropriately instructed were able to self-administer intravenous infusions.[9] Seventy-five percent of our patients were able to return to work and to school, therefore leading productive lives while they were receiving parenteral antibiotic therapy for their infection.[9]

FIGURE 1. Total number of patients treated at Intracare

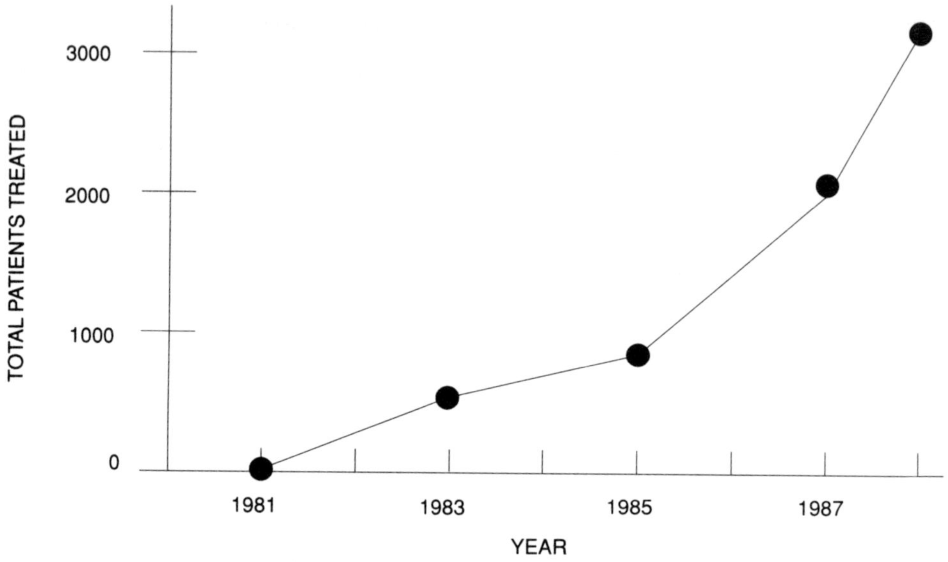

1988	3200
1987	2096
1985	935
1983	500

From the origins of the Intracare clinic concept in 1981, we have grown to the point where to date we have treated more than 3,200 patients (Figure 1). It is interesting to note that, while the numbers of patients have increased, the types of infections treated have remained constant. These are listed in order of frequency in Table III. Of our first 3,247 patients, 38% were treated for bone and joint infections; 23% for infections of skin and of skin structure; 13% for infections of the respiratory tract; 8% for complicated infections of the urinary tract; 3% for chronic pelvic inflammatory disease; and 2% for endocarditis.

TABLE III. Infections treated in outpatients

Diagnosis	Number of Cases
Osteomyelitis	307
Wound infection	138
Urinary tract infection	64
Pelvic inflammatory disease (chronic)	55

TABLE III. Continued

Diagnosis	Number of Cases
Septic arthritis or bursitis	52
Sinusitis (chronic)	51
Cellulitis	49
Intra-abdominal abscess	47
Mucocutaneous herpes simplex infection	38
Otitis media (chronic)	31
Endocarditis	26
Pneumonitis	25
Septicemia	21
Herpes zoster	14
Typhoid fever	7
Dental infection	6
CMV retinitis	2
Meningitis	2
Total	**935**

Of the first 3,247 patients treated, ceftriaxone and cefazolin were used in approximately one-third of the cases (Table IV.). Because of the recent increases in the number of methicillin-resistant *Staphylococcus aureus* and *Staphylococcus epidermidis* infections, we have used vancomycin with increased frequency. Because of potency and lack of side effects it is expected that fluoroquinolones, like ciprofloxacin, will eliminate the need for parenteral therapy in several groups of patients, particularly those with gram-negative bacillary osteomyelitis or chronic skin structure infections. In fact, based upon data presented in later chapters in this book, there has been impressive outpatient utilization of ciprofloxacin for infections that previously would have required inpatient care.

TABLE IV. Drugs administered to outpatients

Drugs	Number of Cases
Cefazolin	216
Ceftriaxone	129
Cefoperazone	104
Tobramycin	90
Clindamycin	74
Gentamicin	62
Acyclovir	52
Chloramphenicol	44
Vancomycin	32
Cefuroxime	31
Penicillin	22
Moxalactam	22
Amphotericin	13
Miscellaneous	44
Total	**935**

DEVELOPMENT OF QUALITY CONTROL

While it is expected that the administration of ambulatory antibiotic therapy will be valued at $15 billion in 1991,[10] there still is a lack of quality assurance for the various systems. Important issues that need to be addressed include the drop-out rate of those who have entered the program, adverse drug reactions, medication errors, intravenous device complications, patient satisfaction and the efficacy of therapy. Comparisons between costs for outpatient versus inpatient ambulatory therapy can be made quite easily. For example, it is calculated that in our first 3,247 patients, $24.4 million in hospitalization costs were saved because of the employment of ambulatory antibiotic therapy.[11] However, comparative efficacy evaluations between inpatient and outpatient populations receiving such therapy are lacking. In fact, there have been only a few efficacy evaluations since the early work by Antoniskis and colleagues,[3] who did not show statistically significant results because of small numbers of patients.

We evaluated a segment of our population treated for osteomyelitis and compared these patients to historical controls. For controls data collated by Waldvogel and colleagues[12] was used. They reported efficacy rates of 82% for acute hematogenous osteomyelitis, 60% for acute osteomyelitis due to a contiguous septic focus, 25% for chronic osteomyelitis due to a contiguous septic focus, and 10% for osteomyelitis (both acute and chronic) complicated by vascular insufficiency. We[13] reviewed results in 427 cases of osteomyelitis treated on an outpatient basis. Osteomyelitis due to hematogenous dissemination accounted for 64 cases, osteomyelitis complicated by vascular insufficiency accounted for 106 cases, and osteomyelitis due to a contiguous septic focus for 257 cases. Our efficacy rates were very similar to the Waldvogel rates, i.e., 88% cure rate for osteomyelitis caused by hematogenous dissemination, 70% for acute osteomyelitis caused by a contiguous septic focus, 27% for chronic osteomyelitis acquired from a contiguous septic focus, and 28% for both acute and chronic cases of osteomyelitis complicated by vascular insufficiency. These data (Table V.) suggest that intravenous antibiotic therapy in an outpatient setting is as efficacious as therapy in an inpatient setting, and more cost-effective.

TABLE V. Cure rates of inpatient and outpatient therapy of osteomyelitis (from references 12 and 13)

Types of Osteomyelitis	Mass. General Hospital	Intracare
Acute Hematogenous	82%	88%
Acute Contiguous Focus	60%	70%
Chronic Contiguous Focus	25%	27%
Vascular Insufficiency	10%	28%

THE FUTURE

With the present demands to reduce hospitalization costs, it is clear that there is tremendous pressure to discharge patients from the hospital as early as possible. At the same time, the number of hospital beds is certainly not growing and may be contracting. These trends complicate the care of our aging population, a group in which disease is more prevalent and more severe. Thus, there may be a genuine squeeze on the hospitalization of patients that will require a triage system wherein only the most ill can be hospitalized. I have in the past predicted that these pressures will force out the present medical/surgical inpatients to day-care centers that I have called protohospitals.[11] These protohospitals will be able to offer the same diagnostic and therapeutic techniques that conventional present day hospitals provide, but they will be streamlined into more cost-effective machines. I believe that Intracare and other ambulatory clinic models treating infectious disease patients in an outpatient setting are the forerunners of the protohospital.

REFERENCES

1. Spiegel AD. Home Health Care (1987, Rynd Communications, Owings Mill, MD).
2. Rucker RW, Harrison GM. Outpatient intravenous medications in the management of cystic fibrosis. Pediatrics 1974; 54:358-60.
3. Antoniskis A, Anderson BC, Van Volkinburg EJ, et al. Feasibility of outpatient self-administration of parenteral antibiotics. West J Med 1978;128:203-6.
4. Stiver HG, Telford GO, Massey AM, et al. Intravenous antibiotic therapy at home. Ann Intern Med 1978;89:690-3.
5. Kind AC, Williams DN, Persons G, et al. Intravenous antibiotic therapy at home. Arch Intern Med 1979;139:413-5.
6. Poretz DM, Eron LJ, Goldenberg RI, et al. Intravenous antibiotic therapy in an outpatient setting. JAMA 1982;248:336-9.
7. Rehm SJ, Weinstein AJ. Home intravenous antibiotic therapy: a team approach. Ann Intern Med 1983;99:388-92.
8. Eisenberg JM, Kitz DS. Savings from outpatient antibiotic therapy for osteomyelitis. Economic analysis of a therapeutic strategy. JAMA 1986;255:1584-8.
9. Poretz DM, Woolard D, Eron LJ, et al. Outpatient use of ceftriaxone: a cost benefit analysis. Am J Med 1984; 77(4c):77-83.
10. Eron LJ. Intravenous antibiotic administration in outpatient settings. J Infect Dis 1985; 14(Vol 10):4-9.
11. Eron LJ. Outpatient intravenous antibiotic therapy. Hospital Formulary 1988;23:440-7.
12. Waldvogel FA, Medoff G, Swartz MN. Osteomyelitis: a review of clinical features, therapeutic considerations, and unusual aspects. N Engl J Med 1970;282:198-206, 260-6, 316-22.
13. Ingram C, Eron LJ, Alder M, et al. Antibiotic therapy of osteomyelitis in outpatients. Med Clin North Am 1988; 72:723-38.

CHAPTER 2

Patient-Physician Communications and Adherence

Irwin M. Rosenstock, Ph.D.
Long Beach, CA

INTRODUCTION

This chapter focuses on factors that influence patients to comply with medical advice, with particular reference to the role of patient-physician relationships. While the terms compliance and adherence have sometimes been used in slightly different ways, they are used interchangeably in this chapter. In addition, the term "patient-physician communication" is used generally to include face-to-face professional interactions between clients and health providers of all kinds.

To provide a setting for a discussion of influential factors affecting compliance, it is important first to consider the scope of non-compliance, the rational basis for failure to comply and problems in measuring compliance.

Also, while this book is devoted to recent advances in antimicrobial therapies, the literature on compliance does not reveal different kinds of determinants for different kinds of health problems, although the weights of various factors may differ across various types of diseases. Accordingly, the review of literature on compliance will include studies of compliance directed toward control of chronic disease as well as compliance with regimens of antimicrobial therapy.

MAGNITUDE AND SCOPE OF THE COMPLIANCE PROBLEM

Although many of the diseases that currently plague the human species are preventable or treatable, not all of these are currently being prevented or treated. Deaths from communicable diseases for which there are simple, effective immunizations still occur; sexually transmitted disease is a perennial and growing problem. Diseases of nutritional deficiency still take a major toll in the health and vitality of large numbers of Americans, and millions follow lifestyle patterns known to be deleterious to health. A major factor in the gap between the possibilities for disease prevention and control and actual health outcomes is the fact that health recommendations are not systematically followed.

In the recent past, particularly since the advent of antimicrobial agents, there has been a rapid growth of interest in the issue of patient compliance or adherence to medical regimens. "The gap," noted one investigator, "between the therapy prescribed by the physician and the therapy actually taken by the patient is distressingly wide for self-administered regimens."[1]

While estimates of adherence to recommendations vary widely, there is firm evidence that substantial nonadherence occurs in almost every circumstance where some form of self-administration is involved. An early landmark analysis by Sackett,[1] which averaged results over many studies of medication administration, suggested that (1) 50% of patients do not take prescribed medications in accordance with instructions, (2) 20% to 40% of clients do not come in for recommended immunizations, (3) one third of patients observed across a number of studies fail to take any of their prescribed medications, one-third take almost all, with the remaining third scattered in between, and (4) scheduled appointments for treatment are missed 20% to 50% of the time. Subsequent reviews, some as recent as 1987, present an equally stark picture of widespread failure of patients to follow professional health advice.[2-4]

The existence of such substantial failure to comply with health recommendations often surprises health workers, who may assume that good compliance is the norm. If a therapy is worthwhile, which in itself may be an untested assumption,[5] then its benefits cannot be gained in the absence of adherence. Moreover, the efficacy of some drugs depends on maintenance of proper blood levels, which cannot be achieved if dosing is erratic or incomplete. One possible ramification of noncompliance is that if a course of therapy seems ineffective, the therapist may try more heroic measures or shift treatment without knowing whether the recommended regimen has been followed adequately. Studies of physicians' ability to predict compliance in patients reveal only chance levels of accuracy.[6] Therefore, it is apparent that professionals are often unaware of the extent and magnitude of nonadherence.

A further problem created by variations in adherence levels relates to procedures for establishing efficacy of therapeutic maneuvers. In trials that test the efficacy of a medication, proper comparison of treated with untreated groups or of varying dosage levels assumes that the treatment actually takes place. Incomplete compliance, especially if its extent is not fully known, can have a devastating effect, both upon the sample-size requirements for showing real differences between treatment and control groups and upon the ability to conclude that treatments have clinically significant effects.

In light of the statistics on non-compliance one might be tempted to assume a popular disinterest in, or even an aversion to, health-related activity. But any interpretation of public disinterest in health is quickly dispelled by the enormous market for over-the-counter medications, medical appliances, books about "wellness" and "selfcare," special foods, exercise videos, and the like. As Sir William Osler observed, "The desire to take medicine is perhaps the greatest feature which distinguishes man from animals."[7]

The difficulty lies neither in arousing people's interest in health matters nor in overcoming some widespread reluctance to acknowledge illness or to attempt cure, but rather in persuading individuals to adopt those regimens specified by health professionals.

A RATIONAL BASIS FOR NON-COMPLIANCE

As indicated, the existence of poor compliance levels often surprises health workers to whom such behavior appears counter-intuitive. When clinicians become aware of non-compliance, they tend to blame it on the patient's personality and express little sympathy for the uncooperative patient.[8] However, the compliance-related attitudes and performance of clinicians are not unlike those of patients in general.[9,10]

By the time the average person reaches adulthood, he or she is likely to have experienced many successes and many failures with the outcomes of medical recommendations. Most people have encountered or experienced circumstances wherein faithful adherence to a regimen does not yield the desired outcome: the diagnosis may have been incorrect; the prescribed therapy may have been incorrect (or inadequate, or inefficacious); the patient may not have responded to a particular treatment. The lesson learned by the individual is this: sometimes, even if you do everything the doctor tells you to do, you still don't get well. Similar, but opposite, learning experiences are encountered in which the patient recovers despite poor compliance. Again, the wrong diagnosis may have been made or the condition may have been self-limiting.

Further, many persons are wary of the possible adverse consequences of different medications and therapies. Individuals are continually exposed by the mass media to controversies, contradictions, and often reversals with regard to public health and medical care recommendations (e.g., the perennial debates about the pros and cons of obtaining various influenza immunizations, of sharply altering dietary patterns, or of achieving "ideal" body weight). One is impressed by the contemporary relevance of Chapin's comment, made in 1915, that

> the opprobrium of our art is that preventive medicine, like its other branches, has taught much that has had to be unlearned. We ought not to be surprised that people do not believe all we say, and often fail to take us seriously. If their memories were better, they would trust us even less.[11]

When people are ill, the presence of symptoms forms a focal event for reacting to advice,[12] and where action is directed toward relief of symptoms, recommendations are usually followed more faithfully.[6] The other side of the coin is that premature termination of a regimen is often associated with the disappearance of symptoms. In one study of children given penicillin for an acute infection, mothers most frequently cited remission of symptoms as the reason for stopping the medication.[13]

It should be emphasized that it is the individual's interpretation of symptoms, not the physician's interpretation that provides the key to understanding the role of symptoms in behavior. Symptom occurrence is ubiquitous and most symptoms are dealt with outside the medical care system.[14] It is, of course, well known that people may not act on apparently severe symptoms, a situation illustrated by the research on delay in seeking care.[15]

MEASURING COMPLIANCE

An important issue in the study of the fate of professional recommendations is measuring the behaviors involved. As in most areas of human behavior, there are difficulties associated with making the concepts of interest operational.

An individual's public actions are relatively simple to record. Thus, assessment of appointment keeping or of an immunization may be straightforward; however, even in these situations not all visits and services are recorded. Use of services over periods of time or for specific purposes is somewhat more difficult to measure, and losses occur because people change sources of care or because record systems are always less complete and accurate than might be imagined. Studies of populations utilizing several sources of care make the use of records more difficult; so do nonstandardized and haphazard record systems.

Private behaviors not subject to regular entry in medical records pose measurement problems of still greater magnitude. While there is, now, a considerable literature on assessment of medication behavior,[16] measures vary in their apparent validity and directness. Ideally, one would like to observe the extent to which patients actually consume prescribed drugs. Because that is not possible in the outpatient setting, investigators have utilized pill counts or assessments of physiological traces of drugs through blood or urine tests. Pill counts are not easy to do and pose a series of problems. For example, medications are not always kept in their original containers, supplies are divided up, kept in several places, even shared with spouses, and containers are not returned on request; moreover, frankly acknowledged pill counting is probably reactive, in that compliance may well increase if people believe they will be studied. Physiological assessments have advantages but may be costly and, again, may alter behavior if patients know they are going to be tested. In addition, the amount of a drug present in the body is dependent on its pattern of uptake and physical characteristics of the individual, so that variation occurs in blood levels even under conditions of perfect compliance.

Many investigators rely on self-report by the patient – an obvious source of information but one that is subject to several sources of invalidity.[16] Self-report may yield overestimates of adherence to recommendations,[17] although some studies of medication adherence in which self-report was compared with other methods of assessment have yielded accurate results.[18,19] Recent evidence indicates that self-report of compliance is more accurate when the client is led to believe that the individual report will be checked against a biological marker.[20]

The other referent of the concept of adherence – the professional recommendation – should not be forgotten. Medical advice dispensed to patients includes: the objective recommendation; the recorded advice, if any; what is reported by the patient; and what is reported by the health professional. Ideally, there should be a close match among these; in fact, they do not always correspond well.[21] Ley and Spellman[22] have shown that the patient typically remembers only a fraction of the advice given. Hulka's work[21] has concentrated on the congruence between the reports of patient and physician as it affects compliance. In considering any type of professional-lay communication, there is always a question of how it is initially perceived and subsequently recalled by a patient.

PSYCHOSOCIAL FACTORS AND COMPLIANCE

Let us consider relationships of adherence behaviors to personal, social, and situational variables. Haynes[6] reviewed factors associated with compliance to medical regimens, covering some 185 original research reports, and summarized a variety of factors: demographic characteristics of patients; features of the disease, regimen and therapeutic source; aspects of patient-physician interaction; and sociobehavioral characteristics of patients. He concludes that only a small number of variables have demonstrated consistent relationships with patient adherence. Among these factors – all of which are associated with lower rates of compliance –

are: the complexity, duration, and amount of change involved in the regimen itself; inconveniences associated with operation of clinics; inadequate supervision by professionals; patient dissatisfaction; certain kinds of health beliefs; non-compliance with other regimens; and family instability. This summary is noteworthy more for what it does not include than for what it does include – namely, the many variables studied that have not yielded consistent relationships with adherence across different situations and regimens, such as demographic factors, personality characteristics, health knowledge, health status, and social norms.

Other reviewers have supported the conclusions of Haynes that there are no consistent associations between compliance and ordinary social characteristics of patients, such as age, sex, and education.[23,24]

The term "defaulter" has occurred in the literature of compliance, its connotation being that of a peculiar constellation of enduring personal traits that make the individual non-compliant. However, there is by now widespread agreement that the existence of the defaulting patient is a myth.[25] Although a number of personality-like measures have been utilized in studies of compliance, they have not been successful in predicting compliance. Moreover, patients will frequently comply with some elements of a regimen while rejecting other elements, and a given patient may comply with a regimen on one occasion, or for one condition, yet fail to comply with a regimen for another condition or on another occasion.

It might be suspected that level of knowledge would be associated with level of adherence. However, studies have not found consistent associations between general medical knowledge and adherence.[6] Provision of information about the nature of illness and its treatment at an abstract level has generally not increased adherence.[6]

A different kind of "knowledge" does appear related to compliance – namely, the extent to which the patient knows what behavior the regimen requires and how and when to perform this behavior. A number of studies have found that possession of this kind of information relates positively to adherence.[13,21] In one study of a low-income population,[26] about 50% of the patients could not correctly report how long they were supposed to continue on their medications; about 25% did not know what dosage was prescribed; about 15% could not report the prescribed frequency with which they were to take their medications; about 15% thought that drugs marked PRN were to be taken regularly; and about 20% could not identify the purpose of each drug they were taking. When these conditions were examined in relation to compliance, it was found that about 70% of those who correctly recalled their physician's instructions were adhering to their regimen, but only 15% of patients complied if they made one or more mistakes in reporting facts about their regimen.

It is worth noting that as many as half the physician's statements are forgotten by the patient almost immediately;[27] therefore, whenever possible, understandable, written instructions should be provided to reinforce the oral communication.

Reduced adherence occurs when the regimen is complex, of long duration, inconvenient, or expensive.[6,28] For example, in one study medication errors were less than 15% when only one drug was prescribed, increased to 25% when two or three drugs were taken, and exceeded 35% when five or more drugs were taken.[29]

CLIENT HEALTH BELIEFS

During the past two decades, considerable attention has been given to efforts to explain patient non-compliance as a problem in health-related decision making, in which the individual is guided by personal attitudes and beliefs. Considerable empirical research has accumulated supporting what is now labeled the Health Belief Model (HBM), which suggests that whether an individual will follow professional advice often depends on four factors:

(1) *health motivation*, i.e., the degree of interest in, and concern about, health matters in general;

(2) *perceived susceptibility* or vulnerability (or resusceptibility) to the particular illness (or to its sequelae). Note that perceived-susceptibility includes acceptance of the diagnosis;

(3) *perceived severity* concerning the probable seriousness of the physical and social consequences of the untreated illness; and

(4) *perceived benefits and costs* of complying with the advocated health behavior. The issue here is how effective the treatment is expected to be weighed against a subjective estimate of the costs or barriers that might be involved in undertaking the recommended action. Costs or barriers include financial expense, physical and/or emotional discomfort, inconvenience, and the possibility of adverse side effects.[30]

Although the HBM was originally developed to account for preventive health actions,[31,32] it has been employed successfully to explain compliance behavior in seeking a diagnosis and in following prescribed medication, diet, and other regimens,[33-39] and even as a predictor of general clinic utilization.[40,41] Of the patient health beliefs described above, the one that most often puzzles practitioners is the patient's failure to accept a diagnosis: why would a person seek out and subject himself or herself to costly, inconvenient expert examination and consultation and then reject that professional's conclusions?

At least three kinds of situations can undermine belief in diagnosis. First, the patient may possess powerful, well-defined (albeit scientifically erroneous) health beliefs that conflict with the physician's assessment of the problem. Some people may believe that they or their children cannot contract a particular disease because "it does not run in the family." Such beliefs may have multiple origins (e.g., from cultural subgroups, parental beliefs, prior experiences with an illness, misinterpretation of factual information, or acceptance of information from nonmedical sources).

Second, incidents may occur during the history-taking or physical workup that weaken the patient's confidence in the diagnosis (e.g., where the physician appears to pay insufficient attention to the presented complaint). There is also the difficulty that many patients are not totally candid with their physicians about everything worrying or bothering them. Patients are often reluctant to trouble a busy professional with minor aches and concerns, or the symptoms may be too embarrassing to discuss, or social distance between the professional and the lay patient may encourage reticence; nonetheless, these problems and symptoms continue to worry the patient. Thus, if the physician arrives at a diagnosis without identifying the undisclosed concern, the patient may feel that the diagnosis must be inaccurate or incomplete, since it did not include, and therefore did not explain, the problem that was purposely withheld from the physician.

Third, patients sometimes reject a diagnosis that is too painful to accept. They often react initially to a perceived life-threatening illness by denying they have it; a similar denial process probably leads to delay in seeking care for symptoms that the patient believes may indicate serious disease. Several studies of health beliefs have shown that people attribute to others a greater risk of contracting illnesses than they estimate for themselves.[42]

The degree to which providers can modify patients' health beliefs is difficult to assess. Nonetheless, research has demonstrated that beliefs in susceptibility, severity, benefits and costs can be altered.[43,44] Thus, by learning which of these beliefs is below a level presumed necessary for good adherence, the provider can tailor interventions to suit the unique needs of each client. Jenkins[45] has suggested that attention to the beliefs in the HBM during the diagnostic phase will identify what content should be emphasized in teaching about the specific diseases to be prevented or treated and the specific health behaviors to be encouraged. *Are they beliefs about susceptibility or about severity? Is it failure to believe the treatment will be effective? Are the costs believed to be too high?*

Of course, knowing why many patients do not follow their regimens does not imply any particular strategy for changing the behavior. Sometimes merely providing corrective, factual information will prove sufficient; in other cases, stronger interventions may be needed, including motive-arousing appeals to pride or to parental or family responsibilities, or recommendations from highly credible sources of information.

It is perhaps worth noting that fear-arousal techniques have often been employed to change health-related attitudes and behaviors, and these techniques often do have a positive influence on compliance.[46,47] However, fear-arousal must be used carefully; while low levels of concern about the threat of some illness or condition are not likely to motivate action, too much fear can inhibit adaptive behavior. In general, the literature suggests that fear appeals are most effective under two conditions: (1) when they are used with persons who have little or no initial concern with a particular health problem; and, equally important, (2) when they are accompanied by specific behavioral recommendations that the patient can easily and quickly initiate to reduce the threat.[48]

A recent review of research on the HBM[49] summarized the results of 46 studies. Overall, these investigations provide substantial evidence of the importance of health beliefs in understanding patient adherence.

Recent research has demonstrated the importance of one explanatory variable that should be added to the HBM. Bandura[50] has developed the concept of self-efficacy, which he defines as "the conviction that one can successfully execute the behavior required to produce (the) outcomes." No behavior will be undertaken unless the individual believes himself or herself capable of doing it. Bandura suggests ways of increasing self-efficacy. For example, patients may be encouraged to achieve success by mastering elements of a complex regimen one at a time, they may be influenced by exposure to others who have mastered a regimen, or their initial efforts may be encouraged and reinforced by praise and encouragement given by the doctor or by others. Particularly where recommended behavior is complex and of long duration, self-efficacy is of critical importance to compliance.[51,52]

In considering interventions to enhance compliance, one should first try possible modifications in characteristics of the medical regimen. Regimens can be made less complex by: (1) avoiding the routine prescription of nonessential medicine, unnecessary doses, or variations in scheduling; (2) emphasizing the necessity of adherence to particularly critical aspects of the treatment (prioritizing the regimen); (3) breaking the treatment plan into less complex stages that can be implemented sequentially (graduated regimen implementation); and (4) minimizing both inconvenience and forgetfulness by matching the regimen schedule to the patient's regular daily activities, that is, tailoring the regimen.[20,43,53,54] Short-term therapy, or at least the perception of it, can be accomplished by scheduling follow-up visits in quick succession when progress can be shown, thus giving the patient a feeling of accomplishment and a sense of the treatment's importance.[28]

THE PATIENT-PHYSICIAN RELATIONSHIP AND COMPLIANCE

The quality of the relationship between patient and physician is crucial to the patient's understanding of the disease and its treatment and to patient's satisfaction and compliance.[19,55] Features and effects of the system through which patients interact with professionals have a marked influence on outcomes. It has been demonstrated that the language and concepts of the medical field are not widely understood.[56] Not only are many of the technical words foreign to patients, but also many commonly used bits of advice go misunderstood. Recommendations such as "reduce salt intake" or "take the medicine on an empty stomach" may be misinterpreted. McKinlay[57] demonstrated that patients' understanding of terms commonly used by physicians varies considerably; and in addition, he found that physicians use terminology that they themselves believe is not understood by patients. Even in the interpretation of instructions on prescriptions, researchers have found considerable ambiguity.[58] In a sample of patients who were asked to interpret instructions on drug labels, only 36% correctly stated what "every six hours" means. Interpretations varied considerably on what is meant by "evening" and by "with meals."

The doctor-patient relationship may be viewed from two distinct but interactive perspectives, the *affective* or emotional interaction and the *coqnitive* or intellectual interaction. Both perspectives influence patient compliance.

Affective Perspective

Following an evaluation of the affective level, Coe and Wessens[59] suggested that numerous aspects of the physician-patient interaction, such as impersonality and brevity of encounter, negatively affect patient behavior, and more recent reviews support their conclusions.[2,23,60] Lack of communication, particularly of an emotional nature, is usually seen as the problem. Davis[61] found that failure of patients to comply with doctors' advice often depends on unrelieved tension in the interaction in which the physician is formal, rejecting, or controlling, disagrees with the patient, or interviews the patient at length without later providing feedback. Francis and colleagues[19] report that a mother's compliance with a regimen prescribed for her child is better when she is satisfied with the initial contact, regards the physician as friendly, and feels that the doctor understood the complaint. Further, these investigators found that key factors in non-compliance included the extent to which patients' expectations from the medical visit were left unmet, lack of warmth in the doctor-patient relationship, and failure by the mother to receive an explanation of the diagnosis and cause of the child's illness.

The provider's orientation toward the patient and desire to influence patient compliance are important factors. Schulman[62] found, for instance, that patients who received medical care oriented towards them as active participants in the treatment process were significantly more likely than other patients to comply with medical advice and to display more favorable cognitive and behavioral responses in the management of their illnesses.

Other investigations have also shown positive correlations between compliance and patient satisfaction with the visit, the therapist, or the clinic, including perceptions of convenience and of waiting times before and during appointments.[23] Compliance is greater when patients feel their expectations have been fulfilled, when the physician elicits and respects patients' concerns and provides responsive information about their condition and progress, and when sincere concern and sympathy are shown.

Cognitive Perspective

Turning to the cognitive aspects of the relationship, Ley[63] describes a model of doctor-patient communication which emphasizes its effects on patient understanding, memory, satisfaction and compliance. Ley reminds us that patients frequently fail to understand what they are told and frequently and quickly forget much of what they have understood. His review shows that between 35% and 92% of patients will not understand information given to them and about 40% of this information will soon be forgotten. It is therefore no surprise that about one-third of patients are dissatisfied with doctor-patient communication. Furthermore, satisfaction is positively associated with compliance. If patient comprehension and memory could be improved, satisfaction and compliance would also be increased. Ley estimates that compliance rates could reach 72% if all three variables in his cognitive model - comprehension, memory and satisfaction – increased only modestly; and he provides suggestions for improving understanding and memory.[63]

Ley[63] reports the positive effects of physician awareness of the adherence problem in a controlled trial by Inui and associates.[64] In this study, one of two groups of physicians was given special tutorials (one hour to two hours in length), the content of which emphasized both compliance difficulties of patients with hypertension and possible strategies for altering patient beliefs and behaviors (based on the health belief dimensions described earlier in this chapter). After only a single session, physicians in the experimental group were observed to spend a greater proportion of clinic-visit time on patient teaching, and their patients later exhibited higher levels of knowledge and appropriate beliefs about hypertension and its treatment; moreover, the patients of tutored physicians were subsequently more compliant with the treatment regimen and demonstrated better blood pressure control than did other patients.

Ley[63] also reports that general practitioners who followed suggestions for improving communication increased the patients' recall of what they were told. The rationale for altering patients' behavior in the consultation is that patients are often too diffident to ask questions, even when they know that clarification is needed, or have worries about which they would like reassurance. Roter[65] found that teaching patients to request information they desired from their physicians led to lowered drop-out from clinic attendance.

The provision of written information is still another possibility for increasing patients' knowledge.[66] Of course, as indicated earlier in this chapter, written information must be at a readability level that is understandable to the patient.

It was earlier stated that the affective and cognitive elements of the patient-physician communication are interactive. Quite clearly the ability to understand and to remember professional communications enhances patient satisfaction and that satisfaction, in turn, enhances compliance. But it is also true that the friendly and interested physician communicates more effectively with patients, thus increasing initial understanding and memory and compliance.[62] The message to be learned is that health care providers would be well advised to attend both to the emotional and to the intellectual aspects of their interactions with patients.

The importance of affective and cognitive elements of the doctor-patient relationship for compliance poses a challenge to clinicians and to medical educators. Historically, health care providers, particularly physicians, have been trained for a relationship in which the physician is active and the patient is passive. The physician prescribes and the patient follows doctor's orders. Szasz and Hollender[67] contrast this traditional form of relationship with a mutual participatory mode in which an active partnership between physician and patient is employed to assist patients to help themselves. Coleman's[60] suggestion that physicians can enhance compliance by demonstrating compassion, by effective communications, by activating patient self-motivation and by sharing responsibility with the patient reflects the mutual participatory mode, as does Schulman's[62] concept of active patient orientation.

CHALLENGE FOR THE FUTURE

The challenge is to teach health-care providers to adopt a mutual participatory mode of relationship during a time in history when merely keeping up with advances in technology can occupy one full-time.

The Physician

It is interesting to note, however, that in the studies of Cockburn and colleagues,[53,54] younger general practitioners, with fewer years in practice elicited higher compliance rates for antibiotic treatment among a group of 233 Welsh patients than did older practitioners. No explanation of this finding is provided, but it may be suggested that younger doctors are more oriented toward using effective motivational strategies. This is certainly a topic worthy of further study for medical educators.

One way of moving toward a mutual participatory role is through the use of the contingency contract wherein both physician and patient agree on a treatment goal and a time limit for its achievement. These agreements are written down and signed by both parties. Data are now available supporting the provider-client contract as a tool for improving patient adherence.[68,69] Contracts offer a written outline of expected behavior, the involvement of the patient in the decision-making process concerning the regimen and the opportunity to discuss potential problems and solutions with the physician, and a formal commitment to the program from the patient.

Other Health Care Providers

While the main focus in this chapter has been on physicians, other health care providers are important in the provision of instruction, clarification, and reinforcement. Nurses have great potential for exerting an impact on patient health behavior.[70] In addition, recent studies provide strong empirical support for the value of involving pharmacists in attempts to increase patient cooperation with prescribed therapies.[71,72]

As the health care field continues its gradual movement toward group medical practices, some natural divisions of labor may become more feasible than they have been in the past. The physician's role could emphasize diagnosis and therapeutic recommendations while the roles of other health professionals on the team could emphasize educational functions. This is not to say that physicians would give up responsibility for patient education; indeed not. As indicated in much of the previous material, the interaction of the physician with the patient is critical to success. What is suggested, however, is that responsibilities for diagnosis, prescription and education become shared responsibilities with different health care disciplines emphasizing different functions.

The Patient's Family

The emphasis has been on ways in which providers might increase patient compliance through their own efforts. Physicians and other providers may, however, expand their influence by calling on the patient's family to provide assistance and encouragement for patient adherence. Social support seems to be especially important in long-term treatment plans that require continuous action on the part of the patient.[73,74] In one study, those persons who received reinforcement from another family member were more likely to comply in taking medications.[75] The health beliefs of family members and their evaluation of the patient's illness and treatment may influence patient adherence. Compliance may also be altered favorably if the family assumes responsibility for the sick member's care and provides sympathy, support, and encouragement. Success is greatest when the family's normal roles and patterns are compatible with the prescribed regimen for the patient or when the family members are willing to make accommodating changes in their lives and in the family environment.[76] Evidence is thus growing that social support, particularly support provided by the patient's family, plays an important role in influencing compliance. In a review of six studies that examined the relationship between patient adherence and family influence, Haynes[6] concluded that the influence of the family appears to be considerable, with supportive families being associated with greater compliance in five of the six investigations. Dunbar and Stunkard[77] suggest that family support may well be one of the more promising routes for the improvement of adherence.

Although the patient-provider relationship clearly affects adherence, the actual mechanisms by which these influences occur remain obscure and are, therefore, a reasonable target for future research. One consistent finding is that the likelihood of adherence is increased when the patient's expectations of the encounter are matched by what actually occurs.[6,19]

CONCLUSION

The complexities of the compliance problem have been illustrated through discussion of the magnitude of the problem, the failure to find client characteristics that predict compliance, and the complex nature and impact of the provider-patient relationship. On the brighter side, this chapter describes a promising scheme for understanding patient decisions to comply or not to comply with medical advice and proposes simplifications in medical regimens that can do much to improve compliance. Finally, the review suggests particular kinds of *affective* and *cognitive* provider-client interactions that are associated with good levels of compliance.

Based on the material in this chapter, it thus seems possible to optimize patient compliance with health advice by utilizing and building on the research on affective and cognitive components of the patient-physician communication, incorporating the research findings of the Health Belief Model, using other members of the health care team, particularly for patient education, and soliciting the support of members of the patient's family.

REFERENCES

1. Sackett DL. The magnitude of compliance and noncompliance. In: Sackett DL, Haynes RB, eds. Compliance with therapeutic regimens. Baltimore:Johns Hopkins University Press, 1966:8-25.
2. Meichenbaum D, Turk DC. Facilitating treatment adherence. New York:Plenum Publishing Co., 1987.
3. Finney JW, Friman PC, Rapoff MA, et al. Improving compliance with antibiotic regimens for otitis media. Am J Dis Child 1985;139:89-95.
4. Bertakis KD. An application of the health belief model to patient education and compliance: acute otitis media. Family Med 1986;18:347-50.
5. Stimson GV. Obeying doctor's orders: a view from the other side. Soc Sci Med 1974;8:97-104.
6. Haynes RB. A critical review of the 'determinants' of patient compliance with therapeutic regimens. In: Sackett DL, Haynes RB, eds. Compliance with therapeutic regimens. Baltimore: Johns Hopkins University Press, 1976:26-39.
7. Cushing H. Life of Sir William Osler. Oxford: The Clarendon Press, 1925:1:616.
8. Davis MS. Variations in patients' compliance with doctors' orders: analysis of congruence between survey responses and results of empirical investigations. J Behav Med 1966;41:1037-48.
9. Blackwell B, Griffin B, Magill M, et al. Teaching medical students about treatment compliance. J Med Educ 1978;53:672.
10. Shangold MM. The health care of physicians; do as I say and not as I do. J Med Educ 1979;54:668.
11. Chapin CV. Truth in publicity. Am J Publ Health 1915;5:493.

12. Kasl SV, Cobb S. Health behavior, illness behavior, and sick role behavior. Arch Environ Health 1966;12:246-66, 531-54.
13. Becker MH, Drachman RH, Kirscht JP. Predicting mothers' compliance with pediatric medical regimens. J Pediatr 1972;81(4):843-54.
14. Haggerty R, Roghmann K. Noncompliance and self-medication; two neglected aspects of pediatric pharmacology. Pediatr Clin North Am 1972;19:105-15.
15. Antonovsky A, Hartman H. Delay in the detection of cancer: a review of the literature. Health Educ Monogr 1974;2:98-125.
16. Gordis L. Methodologic issues in the measurement of patient compliance. In: Sackett DL, Haynes RB, eds. Compliance with therapeutic regimens. Baltimore: Johns Hopkins University Press, 1976:51-66.
17. Gordis L, Markowitz M, Lilienfield A. The inaccuracy of using interviews to estimate patient reliability in taking medications at home. Med Care 1969;7:49-54.
18. Feinstein A, Wood HF, Epstein JA, et al. A controlled study of three methods of prophylaxis against streptococcal infection in a population of rheumatic children: results of the first three years of study, including methods for evaluating the maintenance of oral prophylaxis. N Engl J Med 1959;260:697-702.
19. Francis W, Korsch BM, Morris MJ. Gaps in doctor-patient communications: patient's response to medical advice. N Engl J Med 1969;280:535-40.
20. Eraker SA, Kirscht JP, Becker MH. Understanding and improving patient compliance. Ann Intern Med 1984;100:258-68.
21. Hulka BS, Cassel JC, Kupper L. Disparities between medications prescribed and consumed among chronic disease patients. In: Lasagna L, ed. Patient compliance. Mt. Kisco, NY:Futura Publishing Company, 1976.
22. Ley P, Spelman MS. Communications in an outpatient setting. Br J Social Clin Psych 1965;4:115-25.
23. Becker MH, Maiman LA. Sociobehavioral determinants of compliance with health and medical care recommendations. Med Care 1975;13(1):10-24.
24. Kasl SV. Socio-psychological characteristics associated with behaviors which reduce cardiovascular risk. In: Enelow AJ, Henderson JB, eds. Applying behavioral science to cardiovascular risk. New York: American Heart Association, 1975.
25. Blackwell B. Drug therapy: patient compliance. N Engl J Med 1973;289:249-53.
26. Svarstad BL. Physician-patient communication and patient conformity with medical advice. In: Mechanic D, ed. The growth of bureaucratic medicine: an inquiry into the dynamics of patient behavior and the organization of medical care. New York: John Wiley and Sons, 1976:220-38.
27. Ley P, Bradshaw PW, Eaves D, et al. A method for increasing patients' recall of information presented by doctors. Psychol Med 1973;3:217.
28. Matthews D, Hingson R. Improving patient compliance: a guide for physicians. Med Clin North Am 1977;61:879.
29. Hulka BS, Kupper LL, Cassell JC, et al. Medication use and misuse: physician-patient discrepancies. J Chron Dis 1975;38:7.
30. Becker MH. The health belief model and personal health behavior. Health Educ Monogr 1974;2:324-473.
31. Becker EH, Kaback MM, Rosenstock IM, et al. Some influences of public participation in a genetic screening program. J Community Health 1975;1:3.
32. Rosenstock IM. Patients' compliance with health regimens. JAMA 1975;234:402.
33. Becker MH. The health belief model and sick role behavior. Health Educ Monogr 1974;2:409.
34. Becker MH, Drachman RH, Kirscht JP. Predicting mothers' compliance with pediatric medical regimens. J Pediatr 1972;81:843.
35. Becker MH, Maiman LA, Kirscht JP, et al. The health belief model and dietary compliance: a field experiment. J Health Soc Behav 1977;18:348.
36. Becker MH, Radium SM, Rosenstock IM, et al. Compliance with a medical regimen for asthma: a test of the health belief model. Publ Health Rep 1978;93:268.

37. Hartman PE, Becker MH. Noncompliance with prescribed regimen among chronic hemodialysis patients: a method of prediction and educational diagnosis. Dialysis Transplant 1978;7:978.
38. Kirscht JP, Rosenstock IM. Patient adherence to antihypertensive medical regimens. J Community Health 1977;3:115.
39. Harris R, Skyler JS, Linn MW, et al. The relationship between the health belief model and compliance as a basis for intervention in diabetes mellitus. In: Psychological aspects of diabetes in children and adolescents, pediatric adolescent endocrinology. Basel: Karger, 1982;10:123-32.
40. Becker MH, Nathanson CA, Drachman RH, et al. Mothers' health beliefs and children's clinic visits: a prospective study. J Community Health 1977;3:125.
41. Leavitt F. The health belief model and utilization of ambulatory care services. Soc Sci Med 1979;13A:105.
42. Kirscht JP, Haefner DP, Kegeles S, et al. A national study of health beliefs. J Health Hum Behav 1966;7:248.
43. Becker MH, Maiman LA, Kirscht JP, et al. The health belief model and dietary compliance: a field experiment. J Health Soc Behav 1977;18:348.
44. Haefner D, Kirscht JP. Motivational and behavioral effects of modifying health beliefs. Publ Health Rep 1970;85:478.
45. Jenkins CD. An approach to the diagnosis and treatment of problems of health related behavior. Int J Health Educ 1979;22(suppl):3.
46. Kirscht JP, Haefner DP. Effects of repeated threatening health communications. Int J Health Educ 1973;16:3.
47. Kirscht JP, Becker MH, Haefner DP, et al. Effects of threatening communications and mothers' health beliefs on weight change in obese children. J Behav Med 1978;1:147.
48. Leventhal H. Fear appeals and persuasion: the differentiation of a motivational construct. Am J Publ Health 1971;61:1208.
49. Janz NK, Becker MH. The health belief model: a decade later. Health Educ Quarterly 1984;11:1.
50. Bandura A. Self-efficacy: toward a unifying theory of behavior change. Psych Rev 1977;84:191.
51. Strecher VJ, DeVellis BM, Becker MH, et al. The role of self-efficacy in achieving health behavior change. Health Educ Quarterly 1986;13:73-92.
52. Rosenstock IM, Strecher VJ, Becker MH. Social learning theory and the health belief model. Health Educ Quarterly 1988;15:175-83.
53. Cockburn J, Reid AL, Bowman JA, et al. Effects of intervention on antibiotic compliance in patients in general practice. Med J Aust 1987;147:324-7.
54. Cockburn J, Gibberd RW, Feid AL, et al. Practice observed. Br Med J 1987;295:814-8.
55. Stiles WB, Putnam SM, Wolf MH, et al. Interaction exchange structure and patient satisfaction with medical interviews. Med Care 1979;17:667.
56. Pratt L, Seligmann A, Reader G. Physicians' views on the level of medical information among patients. Am J Publ Health 1957;47:1277-83.
57. McKinlay J. Who is really ignorant—physician or patient? J Health Soc Behav 1975;16:3-11.
58. Mazzullo J. Methods of improving patient compliance. In: Lasagna L, ed. Patient compliance. Mt. Kisco, NY: Futura Publishing Company, 1976.
59. Coe RM, Wessen A. Social-psychological factors influencing the use of community health resources. Am J Publ Health 1965;44:1024.
60. Coleman VR. Physician behaviour and compliance. J Hypertens 1985;3:Suppl 1:69-71.
61. Davis MS. Variations in patients' compliance with doctors' advice: an empirical analysis of patterns of communication. Am J Publ Health 1968;58:274-88.
62. Schulman BA. Active patient orientation and outcomes in hypertensive treatment: application of a socio-organizational perspective. Med Care 1979;17:267-80.
63. Ley P. Doctor-patient communication: some quantitative estimates of the role of cognitive factors in non-compliance. J Hypertens 1985;3:Suppl 11:51-5.

64. Inui TS, Yourtee EL, Williamson JW. Improved outcomes in hypertension after physician tutorials: a controlled trial. Ann Intern Med 1976;84:646-51.
65. Roter D. Patient participation in the patient-provider interaction. Health Educ Monogr 1977;54:281-306.
66. Ley P, Spelman MS. Communicating with the patient. London: Staples Press, 1979;1-32.
67. Szasz TS, Hollender MM. A contribution to the philosophy of medicine: the basic models of the doctor-patient relationship. Arch Intern Med 1956;97:585-92.
68. Lewis CE, Michnich M. Contracts as a means of improving patient compliance. In: Barofsky, ed. Medication compliance: a behavioral management approach. Thorofare, NJ: Charles B. Slack, 1977:69-75.
69. Janz NK, Becker MH, Hartman PE. Contingency contracting to enhance patient compliance: a review. Patient Educ Counsel 1984;5:165.
70. Marston MV. Nursing management of compliance with medical regimens. In: Barofsky I, ed. Medication compliance: a behavioral management approach. Thorofare, NJ: Charles B. Slack, 1977;139-64.
71. Schwartz MA. The role of the pharmacist in the patient-health team relationship. In: Lasagna L, ed. Patient compliance. Mt. Kisco, NY: Futura Publishing Company, 1976;83-95.
72. Sharpe TR. The pharmacist's potential role as a factor in increasing compliance. In: Barofsky I, ed. Medication compliance: a behavioral management approach. Thorofare, NJ: Charles B. Slack, 1977;133-8.
73. Davis MS. Variations in patients' compliance with doctors' advice: an empirical analysis of patterns of communication. Am J Publ Health 1968;57:274.
74. Caplan R, Robinson EAR, French JRP, et al. Adhering to medical regimens. Ann Arbor: Institute for Social Research, University of Michigan, 1976.
75. Willcox DRC, Gillan R, Hare EH. Do psychiatric outpatients take their drugs? Br Med J 1965;2:790.
76. Becker MH, Green LW. A family approach to compliance with medical treatment: a selective review of the literature. Int J Health Educ 1975;18:173.
77. Dunbar JM, Stunkard AJ. Adherence to diet and drug regimen. In: Levy R, Rifkind B, Dennis B, et al, eds. Nutrition, lipids and coronary heart disease. New York: Raven Press, 1979;391-423.

CHAPTER 3

Treatment of Common Sexually Transmitted Diseases

H. Hunter Handsfield, M.D.
Seattle, Washington

INTRODUCTION

The explosive epidemic of sexually transmitted disease (STD) seen during the past 20 years is perhaps the best example of the influence that social, behavioral and demographic factors can have on the spread of communicable diseases despite the availability of effective therapy. However, recommended treatments for STDs, as for many infections, have changed frequently over the past two decades, and continue to evolve, for several reasons. There have been dramatic changes in the antimicrobial susceptibility of some established STD pathogens (e.g., *Neisseria gonorrhoeae*); previously unrecognized pathogens (e.g., *Chlamydia trachomatis*) have come to be recognized as important contributors to STD morbidity; the viral STDs have grown in frequency even more rapidly than the bacterial ones, and ameliorative chemotherapy has become available for one of these (genital herpes); for some diseases (e.g., syphilis), new information has been uncovered about the limitations of traditional therapies; and the development of new antibiotics and the refinement of older ones have expanded the options for treatment.

Much of this book emphasizes outpatient therapy of infections that heretofore were usually treated in the hospital. With the exception of some complications, however, STDs are routinely diagnosed and treated on an outpatient basis. At least 20 pathogens are regularly transmitted by sexual contact, and these cause 50 or more clinical syndromes. It is beyond the scope of this chapter to review the management of all these conditions. Rather, emphasis is given to the most important STDs likely to be encountered by clinicians in North America. The management of some infections of the female genital tract (e.g., pelvic inflammatory disease, vaginitis syndromes) and infections caused by human immunodeficiency virus (HIV) are discussed in Chapters 4 and 11, respectively.

BASIC PRINCIPLES

Diagnosis

Effective therapy is based on accurate diagnosis. Although most STDs can be suspected and sometimes diagnosed definitively on clinical grounds, many available diagnostic tests for these conditions are underutilized by clinicians. Suspected cases of gonorrhea always should be confirmed by isolation of the organism, because the prevalence of resistant strains now demands that isolates be screened for antimicrobial susceptibility.[1,2] The clinical and epidemiologic criteria for suspecting or diagnosing chlamydial infections are insensitive and nonspecific; without culture or immunochemical identification of *C. trachomatis*, most cases will go undetected or will be inappropriately treated.[3] Many cases of genital herpes can be reliably diagnosed on clinical grounds, but atypical presentations are common, and viral isolation should be attempted for all cases of genital ulceration that are not characteristic of herpes or syphilis.[4,5]

The most common causes of vaginal discharge in sexually active women are mucopurulent cervicitis (the female counterpart of nongonococcal urethritis in men), bacterial vaginosis, trichomoniasis, and candidiasis. Often these conditions cannot be accurately distinguished clinically. Therefore, a combination of microscopic and microbiologic tests on vaginal or cervical secretions should be routine in the offices of clinicians who evaluate such patients. Although the sensitivity, specificity, and clinical role for cytologic, immunochemical or genetic methods to identify genital human papillomavirus (HPV) infections remain undefined, it is clear that visible warts represent a very small portion of the spectrum of HPV infections.[6] Finally, clinicians must maintain a low threshold for the diagnosis of STD; changing sexual mores now place the large majority of young adults at risk for STD for large segments of their lives.

Co-Infections

An important factor in choosing treatment for a sexually transmitted infection is the probability of concurrent infections with other STD pathogens.[7] Historically, this concern focused on the coexistence of incubating or established syphilis with gonorrhea, and this remains an important issue in some subpopulations (e.g., homosexually active men with multiple partners, inner city drug users). However, by far the most common additional STD among heterosexuals with gonorrhea in North America and Europe is genital chlamydial infection. Many studies over two decades have given remarkably consistent results, showing that 15% to 25% of heterosexual men and 30% to 50% of women with gonorrhea are also infected with *C. trachomatis*.[8,9] Women infected with *N. gonorrhoeae* and *C. trachomatis* are at high risk of complications (especially acute salpingitis) in the post-treatment period if treatment does not address the chlamydial infection.

Compliance With Therapy

Historically, much has been made of the presumed unreliability of STD patients, with resulting emphasis on single-dose therapy whenever possible. However, with some exceptions (e.g., the populations served by inner city public clinics), patients with STDs are probably equivalent to most other young adults with respect to compliance with multiple-dose treatment regimens, i.e., variable, but amenable to careful counseling. Therefore, it is important for the clinician and patient to discuss the therapeutic rationale, the importance of compliance, and the potential side effects and appropriate responses to them. Although the few minutes necessary for this process may seem obtrusive in a busy office, it is a good investment in time, because return visits are likely to be prevented. Pharmacists have an important role to play in this process, but this should be viewed as adjunctive to personal counseling by the treating physician.

Management of Sexual Partners

Appropriate management of sexual partners is an integral part of treating patients with STDs. Most STDs are transmitted by persons who are asymptomatic or have minor symptoms that they ignore; it follows that many infected partners will not spontaneously seek medical attention. Failure to assure that the partner is examined and treated often is tantamount to not treating the index case, because of the risk of reinfection. Moreover, untreated partners are likely to continue to spread infection to others. The physician should take specific steps to examine the partner(s) personally or to make a specific referral elsewhere; vague advice to "make sure your partner gets checked" often goes unheeded. Depending on local resources and the specific STD, the local health department may assist in notifying the partner; otherwise, the physician and patient should work together to assure that partners are notified.

It is inappropriate to treat the sexual partners of STD patients without examining them. Compliance of the partner with treatment is likely to be poor in the absence of physician counseling, and the partner is unlikely to fully understand the nature of his or her infection. Co-infections that were not apparent in the index case often are brought to light by examining the partner(s). Without a personal examination, the opportunity is missed to bring additional partners (usually unknown to the index case) to treatment. Moreover, blind prescribing carries a significant medicolegal risk that rises in proportion to the potential toxicity of the treatment, and the practice is to be condemned even in apparently monogamous settings, such as treatment of the husband of a woman with trichomoniasis. There are, however, rare exceptions to this principle. For example, it may be necessary to treat without examination if the partner is in a location remote from medical attention.

GONORRHEA

Antimicrobial Susceptibility

Several factors are involved in selecting an antibiotic for treating gonorrhea. These include pharmacokinetic characteristics, differential efficacy at various anatomic sites of infection, toxicity, convenience of administration (for both patient and clinician), efficacy for coexisting pathogens, and cost. However, the *sine qua non* of course is the activity of the antibiotic against *N. gonorrhoeae.*

Three kinds of resistance to the penicillins and tetracyclines have been documented for *N. gonorrhoeae*[1,2] and are summarized in Table I.

TABLE I. Antibiotic resistance in *Neisseria gonorrhoeae*

1. Beta-Lactamase (penicillinase) producing *N. gonorrhoeae* (PPNG)
   - Plasmid-mediated
   - 4% of gonorrhea in U.S.;
     ≥ 30% in some areas

2. Chromosomally-mediated resistance to penicillin and tetracycline
   - "Lower level" resistance due to gonococcal outer membrane alterations
   - Penicillin or tetracycline MIC ≥ 2 mg/L
   - 10% to 20% of gonorrhea in most geographic areas
   - Accounted for most treatment failures with previously recommended regimens

3. Tetracycline resistance (TRNG)
   - Plasmid-mediated
   - MIC ≥ 16 mg/L
   - Uncommon, but increasing

Chromosomally-mediated resistance results from a series of individually minormutations that reduce the permeability of the organism's outer membrane to these drugs or alter the affinity of naturally occurring penicillin-binding proteins for the penicillins. This resistance was formerly called "low-level" resistance because clinical cure could be affected by raising the treatment dose. However, when the minimal inhibitory concentration (MIC) of an antibiotic reaches a point at which clinical failures are common with the maximum practical doses (penicillin or tetracycline MIC $\geq$ 2.0 mg/L), the strains are considered to have chromosomally-mediated resistance. Figure 1 illustrates the effect of increasing chromosomally-mediated penicillin resistance in the United States over the 45 years since penicillin was first used to treat gonorrhea.

Strains with chromosomally-mediated resistance usually display cross resistance to several antibiotics. Those that are resistant to either penicillin or tetracycline generally have high levels of resistance to the other, as well as to erythromycin. These strains now account for 10% to 20% of gonococci in most areas of North America where they have been sought and are the most common cause of treatment failure in the United States.[2] These strains are especially common in homosexual men with gonorrhea, because the spread of gonorrhea in the homosexual population requires maintenance of a reservoir of rectal infection, and toxic fecal lipids and bile salts in the rectum select for the same genes that confer resistance to antibiotics.[2]

FIGURE 1.

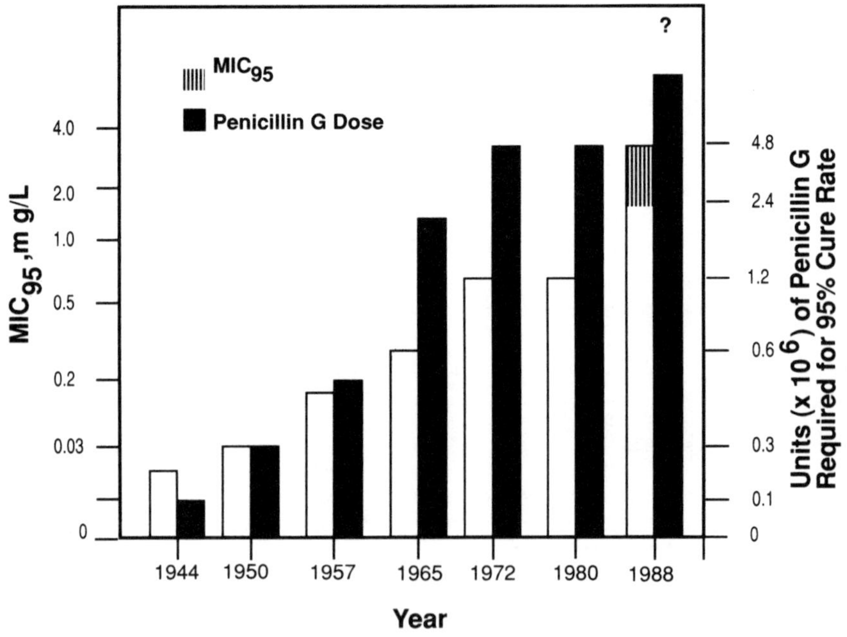

Temporal trends in chromosomally-mediated penicillin resistance in Neisseria gonorrhoeae and penicillin dose in the United States, 1944-1988. MIC_{95} denotes the minimal inhibitory concentration of penicillin required to inhibit 95% of N. gonorrhoeae isolates. The 95% penicillin cure rate refers to the response to single-dose therapy in gonococcal urethritis; various formulations of penicillin are represented, but only aqueous procaine penicillin G (APPG), plus probenecid 1.0 gm orally, was used from 1965 to 1988. The dual shading in the 1988 MIC_{95} bar represents the fact that the penicillin G MIC_{95} varies from 2.0 to 4.0 mg/L in various geographic areas. The dose of APPG plus probenecid that would be required for a 95% cure rate in 1988 is unknown for geographic areas where the MIC_{95} is $\geq$ 4 mg/L.

Strains of gonococci "infected" with a plasmid (extrachromosomal DNA, transmissible between bacteria by conjugation) that confers the ability to produce beta-lactamase (penicillinase) are known as penicillinase-producing *N. gonorrhoeae* (PPNG) strains. First recognized in the Philippines and central Africa in the mid-1970's, PPNG strains rapidly spread worldwide, but they nevertheless remained relatively uncommon in North America for a decade. However, PPNG strains have spread rapidly since 1985 and now account for about 4% of all gonococcal isolates in the United States and up to 40% in some geographic areas.[1]

Still more recently, tetracycline-resistant strains of *N. gonorrhoeae* (TRNG) have appeared.[1,2] These have high level tetracycline resistance (MIC $\geq$ 16 mg/L) due to acquisition of the *Tet-M* plasmid, which also is the genetic basis for tetracycline resistance in some strains of beta-hemolytic streptococci. Although TRNG strains are relatively uncommon in most of North America, they are on the increase and account for several percent of gonococci in some geographic areas (e.g., Baltimore) and occasional isolates in most areas in which they have been sought.

Resistance to penicillin G, both chromosomally-mediated and plasmid-mediated, includes resistance to all of the older penicillins, including ampicillin and amoxicillin. Similarly, tetracycline resistance applies to all drugs of the class, including doxycycline. Fortunately, other therapeutically useful classes of antibiotics have retained excellent activity against *N. gonorrhoeae.* Resistance to spectinomycin, an aminocyclitol antibiotic that has been reserved for 15 years for the treatment of antibiotic-resistant gonorrhea, has been documented, but resistant strains remain very rare in most of the world. The newer cephalosporins (e.g., ceftriaxone) and several other new beta-lactam drugs are beta-lactamase-resistant and thus active against PPNG strains.[1,2,7] These agents also are fully active against strains with chromosomally-mediated resistance, despite the fact that their MICs are slightly higher than for other gonococci.[1,2,7] Finally, the new quinolones (e.g., ciprofloxacin, norfloxacin, enoxacin, ofloxacin, fleroxacin and others) are uniformly highly active against all gonococci.[1,2] However, these drugs are capable of inducing high level resistance in *N. gonorrhoeae in vitro,* and their role in routine gonorrhea therapy is uncertain.

Treatment of Uncomplicated Gonorrhea

The recommended treatment regimens[1,10] for uncomplicated gonorrhea are summarized in Table II.

TABLE II. Recommended treatment of uncomplicated gonorrhea in adults (modified from guidelines of the CDC, from references 1 and 10)

Initial Treatment

Regimen of choice

Ceftriaxone 250 mg intramuscularly (IM)+

Alternative regimens#

Spectinomycin 2.0 gm IM
Cefuroxime axetil 1.0 gm orally plus probenecid 1.0 gm orally
Cefotaxime 1.0 gm IM
Ceftizoxime 1.0 gm IM
Ciprofloxacin 500 mg orally
Norfloxacin 800 mg orally
Amoxicillin 3.0 gm orally plus probenecid 1.0 gm orally **

TABLE II. Continued

Plus Continuing Treatment ++ With

Doxycycline 100 mg orally twice daily for 7 days

or

Tetracycline HCl 500 mg orally four times daily for 7 days

or

Erythromycin 2.0 gm per day orally in divided doses for 7 days##

+ Single doses of 125 mg ceftriaxone have proven effective, but 250 mg is the smallest commercially available unit dose; ceftriaxone is reconstituted in 1% lidocaine

 # Alternative regimens should be restricted to patients who cannot tolerate ceftriaxone, and to those with persistent infection after treatment with ceftriaxone (spectinomycin, ciprofloxacin, or norfloxacin only); most not reliable for pharyngeal gonococcal infection

*** Amoxicillin/probenecid regimen should be used only when the infecting strain of N. gonorrhoeae is known with certainty to be susceptible*

++ Optional for homosexually active men with gonorrhea; see text

Erythromycin should be used only for patients who cannot take doxycycline or tetracycline HCl

Cephalosporins: Ceftriaxone 250 mg intramuscularly (IM) is the initial therapy of choice for all patients in all geographic areas. Ceftriaxone has been shown to be effective in single doses of 125 mg IM, and this dose is employed in some STD clinics;[11] however, 250 mg is the smallest commercially available unit dose and therefore the most convenient for most clinicians.

Ceftriaxone is the only currently recommended single-dose treatment that has been documented to be effective for all potentially infected anatomic sites, including the urethra, cervix, rectum and pharynx. Ceftriaxone is safe and effective in pregnant women, and preliminary data suggest that it effectively aborts incubating syphilis. Treatment with ceftriaxone is convenient and well tolerated, despite the requirement for IM injection; the drug is readily soluble in 1% lidocaine, with which the 0.5 ml or 1.0 ml injection (for 125 mg and 250 mg, respectively) may be given almost painlessly into the deltoid muscle through a 25-gauge needle. In over 10,000 treatment episodes with ceftriaxone at the Seattle-King County Department of Public Health STD Clinics, we have yet to experience serious intolerance or clinically significant toxicity. Although controversy exists concerning the use of cephalosporins in penicillin-allergic patients, cross reactions appear to be uncommon. We use ceftriaxone for patients with penicillin allergy, except for those with clear histories of severe type I reactions (anaphylaxis, rapid-onset urticaria or angioedema, etc.), and have experienced no adverse reactions.

Other cephalosporin antibiotics that have been effective in single doses include cefotaxime 1.0 gm IM, ceftizoxime 500 mg IM, and cefuroxime axetil 1.0 gm orally. Cefuroxime axetil is accompanied by probenecid 1.0 gm orally, to enhance and to prolong cefuroxime blood levels by delaying renal tubular recreation. None of these regimens has been as extensively studied as ceftriaxone, and they are not reliable for pharyngeal gonococcal infection.

Spectinomycin: Spectinomycin 2.0 gm IM is highly effective for anogenital gonorrhea, but even for resistant cases its use has been largely supplanted by ceftriaxone. However, spectinomycin remains the treatment of choice for the rare cases of gonorrhea that persist after ceftriaxone therapy and for patients with allergy or intolerance to both the penicillins and cephalosporins. Administration of spectinomycin is unpleasant for clinician and patient alike, because the drug is administered as a suspension that requires a large bore (18-20 gauge) needle, and the volume injected is large (5 ml).[7] Spectinomycin, unlike the cephalosporins, does not inhibit *Treponema pallidum*. Therefore, patients who receive spectinomycin for gonorrhea should have follow-up serological tests for syphilis 6 to 12 weeks following treatment.

Quinolones: Most of the newer quinolone antibiotics — including ciprofloxacin, norfloxacin, ofloxacin, enoxacin, fleroxacin, and others — have been shown to be effective in single doses for treating uncomplicated anogenital gonorrhea, regardless of the susceptibility of the infecting strain to other antibiotics. An attractive feature of the quinolones is that they are effective when given orally. However, these agents have the potential to induce rapid resistance in *N. gonorrhoeae*. Also, limited numbers of patients have been studied with these drugs, and efficacy for pharyngeal infections is uncertain. Therefore, until more data are available, the quinolones should be used for treating gonorrhea only when the other recommended regimens are contraindicated or otherwise impractical. In these situations, the U.S. Public Health Service recommends single doses of ciprofloxacin 500 mg orally or norfloxacin 800 mg orally.[10] These regimens do not eradicate *C. trachomatis*, despite the fact that most quinolones are active against the organism *in vitro*. These agents are not active against *T. pallidum*, and follow-up serological tests for syphilis are indicated when a quinolone is used to treat gonorrhea.

The penicillins: Aqueous procaine penicillin G (APPG) in a dose of 4.8 million units IM, plus probenecid 1.0 gm orally, formerly was recommended as initial therapy. However, in addition to reduced efficacy because of spreading antimicrobial-resistant gonococci, APPG is the most inconvenient of the previously recommended regimens, requiring two 5 ml IM injections through large bore needles. It is also the most toxic of the readily available regimens, with the potential for acute psychotic reactions due to elevated plasma levels of procaine and for anaphylaxis and other serious allergic reactions.[7] The penicillin era for gonorrhea therapy is over, and there is no legitimate rationale for treatment of any case of gonorrhea with APPG.

Until recently, amoxicillin 3.0 gm orally plus probenecid 1.0 gm orally was the primary initial therapy for uncomplicated gonorrhea,[10] and oral therapy was especially convenient. However, this regimen should never be used unless the patient is known to be infected with a susceptible strain of *N. gonorrhoeae*. Ampicillin 3.5 gm may be substituted for amoxicillin, with identical efficacy.

Supplemental therapy for chlamydial infection: Regardless of the single-dose regimen chosen, heterosexual men and women with gonorrhea should also be treated with doxycycline, 100 mg twice daily, to eradicate coexisting *C. trachomatis* infection.[3,7-10] Tetracycline HCl, 500 mg orally four times daily, also is effective, but doxycycline is better tolerated than tetracycline, and the twice-daily regimen probably enhances compliance. Although historically much more expensive, doxycycline is now available at little more cost than the equivalent tetracycline regimen. The tetracyclines should never be used alone for gonorrhea; there is evidence that widespread use of tetracycline HCl alone in Seattle from 1978 to 1982, because of our concern for chlamydial infection, contributed to a dramatic rise in tetracycline resistance. We failed to consider that there is very little margin between the blood levels of tetracycline achieved with the standard regimen and the maximum tetracycline MIC of gonococci in the community, a situation that is especially conducive to the selection of resistant strains.

Erythromycin is acceptable as a co-treatment if the tetracyclines are contraindicated or not tolerated, although its efficacy for chlamydial infection is less well established than that of the tetracyclines. Any of several preparations is acceptable, in a divided dose regimen totalling 2.0 gm per day. The sulfonamides also should be effective for chlamydial infections that coexist with gonorrhea, but the sulfonomides have not been studied extensively for this infection. Neither erythromycin nor the sulfonamides are effective for gonorrhea when used alone.

Special Considerations

Homosexually active men: Ceftriaxone is the sole recommended initial treatment for uncomplicated gonorrhea in homosexual and bisexual men, because adequate coverage for pharyngeal gonorrhea is relatively more important in these patients than in heterosexuals, and spectinomycin and the quinolones are less reliable for pharyngeal gonorrhea. Because of the high prevalence of relatively resistant gonococci in this population, the amoxicillin or procaine penicillin regimens should never be used. Follow-up of initial treatment with doxycycline or tetracycline is optional, because the prevalence of simultaneous chlamydial infection is $\leq$ 10% in these patients, and serious complications due to *C. trachomatis* are relatively uncommon.[7]

Pregnancy: Pregnant women with gonorrhea should be treated with ceftriaxone in a single dose of 250 mg;[10] the 125 mg regimen has not been studied in pregnancy. Spectinomycin also is effective and safe, but the quinolones are contraindicated. Most authorities recommend following ceftriaxone with a seven day to ten day course of erythromycin,[10] because the tetracyclines are contraindicated in pregnant women.

Gonorrhea in children: A detailed discussion of the management of pediatric gonorrhea is beyond the scope of this chapter. Prior to one year of age, most cases result from perinatal transmission from an infected mother; later cases usually are due to sexual abuse. In general, for uncomplicated gonorrhea ceftriaxone should be used in a single dose of 125 mg; this may be increased to 250 mg in children weighing $\geq$ 100 lb (45 kg).[10] Gonococcal ophthalmia is treated with several days of intravenously administered ceftriaxone. There are few data on the prevalence of chlamydial infection in children with gonorrhea, whether perinatally or sexually acquired. The tetracyclines are contraindicated prior to adolescence, and erythromycin has not been well studied in this setting. Accordingly, the usual practice is to obtain a test for chlamydial infection and to withhold specific treatment unless it is positive.

Complicated gonococcal infections: Adults with disseminated gonococcal infection (DGI) should be treated with a seven day to ten day course of ceftriaxone 1.0 gm once daily, either IM or IV.[10] The once-daily ceftriaxone regimen permits outpatient therapy in reliable patients who do not have overt septic gonococcal arthritis or endocarditis. If the infecting organism is documented to be fully susceptible to the penicillins, treatment can be switched to IV penicillin G or ampicillin, or to oral amoxicillin for outpatients without overt septic arthritis. The treatment of gonococcal salpingitis is discussed in Chapter 4; most outpatients are appropriately treated as for uncomplicated gonorrhea, with extension of the duration of doxycycline treatment to ten days. Similarly, the usual outpatient treatment for acute gonococcal or nongonococcal epididymitis is 250 mg ceftriaxone, followed by doxycycline, 100 mg twice daily for ten days.[10]

SYPHILIS

Treponema pallidum remains fully sensitive to very low levels of penicillin, with MICs ≤ 0.03 mg/L, and penicillin G continues as the antibiotic of choice in all stages of syphilis and is the only agent that is clearly documented to give cure rates of over 90%.[10, 12] However, controversy continues about the appropriate dosage and duration of penicillin therapy in some clinical settings. The current recommendations for treatment of syphilis[10,12] are summarized in Table III.

TABLE III. Recommendations for treatment of syphilis
(modified for guidelines of the CDC, from references 10 and 12)

<u>Primary, Secondary and Early Latent Syphilis (less than 1 year duration)</u>

Benzathine penicillin G 2.4 million units intramuscularly (IM) in a single treatment session.

or

Doxycycline 100 mg orally twice daily for 15 days+

or

Tetracycline HCl 500 mg orally four times daily for 15 days+

<u>Syphilis of Over 1 Year Duration Without Central Nervous System Involvement</u>

Benzathino penicillin G 2.4 million IM weekly for three doses (total 7.2 million units)

or

Doxycycline 100 mg orally twice daily for 30 days+

or

Tetracycline HCl 500 mg orally four times daily for 30 days+

<u>Syphilis Involving the Central Nervous System #</u>

<u>Initial Treatment</u>

Aqueous crystalline penicillin G 2-4 million units IV every four hours for 14 days

or

Procaine penicillin G 2.4 million units IM once daily, plus probenecid 500 mg orally four times daily, for 14 days.

<u>Plus Continuing Treatment With</u>

Benzathine penicillin G 2.4 million units IM weekly for three doses (total 7.2 million units)

TABLE III. Continued

For Penicillin-Allergic Patients

Doxycycline 100 mg orally twice daily for 30 days+

+ Tetracycline and doxycycline are distinctly inferior to penicillin and should be used only if there is a definite contraindication to penicillin; patient compliance with therapy is essential

 # Recommended regimens for all symptomatic neurosyphilis and for asymptomatic central nervous system involvement in syphilis over 1 year in duration; some authorities also advocate these regimens for asymptomatic central nervous system involvement in early syphilis

Primary or secondary syphilis responds in ≥ 95% of cases to a single IM dose of 2.4 million units of benzathine penicillin G, which gives treponemacidal blood levels of penicillin for 10 days to 20 days. However, there is evidence that patients with early syphilis who are co-infected with human immunodeficiency virus (HIV) and those with evidence of central nervous system invasion by *T. pallidum* may require more intensive penicillin treatment.[13] All patients with syphilis should be tested for evidence of HIV infection following informed consent and appropriate counseling; those patients who are positive for HIV should undergo lumbar puncture for cerebrospinal fluid (CSF) examination before they are treated,[13] regardless of clinical stage or duration.

CSF examination should be routine for all patients with late syphilis — i.e., greater than one year in duration — regardless of whether they have asymptomatic (latent) infection or clinical evidence of neurological involvement.[10,12] Regardless of the duration of infection, patients with symptomatic central nervous system involvement, as documented by reactive CSF syphilis serology or otherwise unexplained elevations in the CSF leukocyte count or protein level, should receive either IV aqueous penicillin G or IM procaine penicillin G according to the regimens shown in Table III. Neurologically asymptomatic patients should be treated for neurosyphilis if their syphilis is ≥ 1 year in duration. Patients with HIV infection who have CSF abnormalities consistent with central nervous system involvement should be treated as for neurosyphilis, regardless of duration of symptomatology. Patients with late syphilis whose CSF is normal respond well to three doses of benzathine penicillin G, 2.4 million units each dose, at weekly intervals.[10,12,13]

The tetracyclines are active *in vitro* against *T. pallidum*, and 15 days of doxycycline, 100 mg twice daily, or tetracycline HCl, 500 mg four times daily, is effective for early syphilis if taken reliably and if there is no evidence of central nervous system involvement.[10,12] Due to problems with patient compliance, however, and perhaps because of unrecognized central nervous system involvement, the clinical failure rate following tetracycline therapy is substantially higher than that following penicillin therapy. Most patients with syphilis who give histories of allergy to penicillin should be skin tested to confirm their allergic status; doxycycline or tetracycline therapy should be limited to those with positive skin tests. A 30-day course of doxycycline or tetracycline appears to be effective for late syphilis that does not involve the central nervous system,[10] although data are limited.

Most of the tetracyclines do not produce reliable antitreponemal levels in CSF,[12] and most patients with CSF abnormalities should be treated with penicillin even if allergic, using escalating "desensitization" doses in the hospital.[10] Doxycycline, which penetrates the cerebrospinal fluid better than tetracycline HCl, is the best alternative to penicillin. The dose is 100 mg twice daily for 30 days.[10,12] Ceftriaxone in a dose of 0.5 - 1.0 gm IM or IV daily for ten days may also be effective, but this approach is supported only by a single small study and anecdotal reports.[7,12] Erythromycin, formerly considered an option in penicillin-allergic patients, no longer is recommended, due to high clinical failure rates.[12] A possible exception is a pregnant woman who cannot be desensitized and cannot be treated with ceftriaxone.[10]

Adequate follow-up is important for all patients with syphilis. Those with central nervous system involvement should undergo repeat CSF examinations at 3 month to 6 month intervals until normal. The antitreponemal antibody titer, as reflected in the Venereal Disease Research Laboratory (VDRL) test, is a good indicator of therapeutic response, and repeat serological tests for syphilis are indicated one, three, six and 12 months after treatment, regardless of clinical stage. For patients with late syphilis and others whose serologies remain reactive at one year, continued annual tests may be advisable for several years, especially following non-penicillin therapy.

CHLAMYDIAL INFECTION AND RELATED DISORDERS

Chlamydia trachomatis is uniformly susceptible to levels of the tetracyclines readily achieved with oral dosing,[9] and drugs of this class are the treatments of choice (Table IV). Doxycycline, 100 mg orally for seven days, is the preferred regimen.[8-10] Tetracycline HCl, 500 mg four times daily for seven days, is effective, but must be taken on an empty stomach (and therefore causes more gastrointestinal intolerance than doxycycline); in addition, the four times daily regimen probably reduces compliance. The cost of a seven-day regimen of doxycycline is now little more than that of tetracycline, but in some circumstances the lower cost might make tetracycline more favorable. Other tetracycline congeners have no appreciable advantages over doxycycline; minocycline has been studied and is effective, but unpleasant and sometimes disabling vestibular side effects are common. The duration of treatment for chlamydial infections was formerly the subject of some debate, with some authorities recommending courses as long as three weeks. However, persistent infection has never been reliably documented (absent reinfection) following a seven-day course of doxycycline or tetracycline HCl in the recommended doses.[3,9]

TABLE IV. Treatment of uncomplicated *Chlamydia trachomatis* infection in adults (based on guidelines of the CDC, from references 8 and 10)

Doxycycline 100 mg orally twice daily for 7 days
or
Tetracycline HCl 500 mg orally four times daily for 7 days
or
Erythromycin 2.0 gm per day orally in divided doses for 7-10 days+

+ Erythromycin should be used only for patients who cannot tolerate doxycycline or tetracycline

Erythromycin is the primary alternative for patients with contraindications or who cannot tolerate the tetracyclines;[8-10] however controlled experience with erythromycin in the treatment of chlamydial infection is limited. The usual dose is 2.0 gm daily in divided doses (e.g., 500 mg of erythromycin base or stearate four times daily, or 800 mg of erythromycin ethylsuccinate four times daily). Gastrointestinal intolerance commonly limits the use of erythromycin; the usual response to gastrointestinal side effects is to reduce the dose to 1.0 gm daily (e.g., 250 mg of erythromycin base four times daily) and double the duration of therapy (i.e., two to three weeks). However, treatment failure clearly can follow such regimens. Pediatric patients with chlamydial infection should be treated with erythromycin in a dose of 50 mg/kg body weight per day (to a maximum of 2.0 gm per day), in divided doses, for 14 days.[8]

Doxycycline or tetracycline HCl usually is effective, fortunately, in clinical syndromes that mimic chlamydial infection.[14] Only 30% to 50% of cases of nongonococcal urethritis (NGU) and nongonococcal mucopurulent cervicitis are due to *C. trachomatis*, with many of the remainder apparently due to *Ureaplasma urealyticum*. Most cases of NGU and cervicitis initially respond well to the regimens outlined above, although the frequency of persistence or relapse is substantially higher in the non-chlamydial cases, approaching 50% in some series.[14]

The sulfonamides are active *in vitro* against *C. trachomatis*, and although clinical experience is limited, they are indicated when neither the tetracyclines nor erythromycin can be given.[8,9] However, the sulfonamides are inactive against *U. urealyticum* and have little or no clinical value in nonchlamydial NGU or mucopurulent cervicitis. Therefore, the sulfonamides should be reserved for cases in which chlamydial infection has been documented by culture or immunochemical methods. Sulfamethoxazole 1.0 gm twice daily is appropriate.[8] Sulfamethoxazole-trimethoprim 800/160 mg ("double strength" tablet) twice daily for seven to ten days is also a convenient regimen, although the trimethoprim component does not contribute to efficacy.

The lack of other options for chlamydial infection and related syndromes is an inconvenient and sometimes serious problem.[7] Clindamycin has modest activity against *C. trachomatis*, although clinical failures have been reported.[9] High dose amoxicillin (2 to 3 gm per day in divided doses) may be effective in up to 50% of cases.[9] Azithromycin, a long-acting macrolide antibiotic related to erythromycin, causes no gastrointestinal intolerance and is under investigation as a possible alternative to erythromycin and the tetracyclines. The quinolones have modest *in vitro* activity against *C. trachomatis*, but preliminary studies have given variable results, and these agents are not currently recommended for chlamydial infection, NGU, or mucopurulent cervicitis.

Persistent or recurrent NGU is an etiologic and therapeutic enigma.[14] Some cases appear to be caused by tetracycline-resistant strains of *U. urealyticum*. For this reason, and on the basis of clinical experience, the first recourse (after assuring that the patient complied with the first course of therapy and that there has been no sexual re-exposure to an untreated partner) is to administer a seven to ten day course of erythromycin in the dose outlined above.[14] Cases that continue to recur thereafter should be evaluated for bacterial or nonbacterial prostatitis; empiric therapy with three to four week courses of doxycycline (which penetrates well into prostatic tissue and fluid) is sometimes effective.[14] Recurrent nonchlamydial NGU has no clearly defined clinical counterpart in women, and treatment of the sexual partner has not been shown to affect the recurrence rate.[14] It is advisable to examine the partner, but beyond the initial treatment course, repeated treatment probably is not indicated in the absence of clinical evidence of genital tract infection in the partner. Men with recurrent symptoms of scant clear urethral discharge or poorly localized perineal or scrotal pain should be carefully evaluated for objective evidence of urethral or prostatic inflammation before embarking on empiric antibiotic therapy. Many such patients may have psychogenic symptoms or noninfective inflammation of obscure etiology.[14]

CHANCROID

Chancroid is a genital ulcerative condition, often accompanied by suppuration of one or more inguinal lymph nodes, caused by *Haemophilus ducreyi*. Heretofore uncommon in the United States, the incidence of chancroid is increasing in several geographic areas. Chancroid is spread and maintained in populations by prostitutes to a greater degree than most STDs.[5] This may be due to the fact that asymptomatic carriage of *H. ducreyi* is unusual, with almost all infected patients developing genital ulceration. Out of economic necessity, some prostitutes may continue sexual activity despite genital ulcers that would induce others to abstain from intercourse.

Chancroid has been documented as an important factor enhancing the efficiency of transmission of HIV in African prostitutes and their customers. In North America, therefore, chancroid may assume an importance beyond its relatively low incidence because of its potential enhancement of heterosexual transmission of AIDS. This problem is further magnified by the association of chancroid with prostitution and therefore with the use of illicit drugs, another major risk factor for HIV infection. While chancroid may be suspected on clinical and epidemiologic grounds, the mainstay of diagnosis is isolation of *H. ducreyi* from a genital ulcer or lymph node aspirate.[5]

Ampicillin and amoxicillin were formerly used for chancroid, but many strains of *H. ducreyi* carry the same plasmids that code for beta-lactamase in *N. gonorrhoeae* and thus are resistant to the penicillins. Ceftriaxone and erythromycin remain active, and in many areas of the world sulfamethoxazole-trimethoprim also is effective. Historically, chancroid has been treated for seven days to ten days, but recent studies have documented the efficacy of single IM doses of 250 mg ceftriaxone[5,10] (Table V.). However, recent data suggest that single dose therapy has reduced efficacy for chancroid in patients with HIV infection.[10] Erythromycin, 2.0 gm per day in divided doses for seven days, also is effective, and some authorities treat severe cases with both ceftriaxone and erythromycin. The new quinolone antibiotics are highly active against *H. ducreyi*, and preliminary evidence suggests that one or more drugs of this class may have an important future role in chancroid therapy. Fluctuant lymph nodes should be aspirated as necessary, but surgical incision and drainage often delays healing and prolongs morbidity.[5] The sexual partners should be treated with ceftriaxone or erythromycin, regardless of the presence or absence of clinical evidence of infection.[10]

TABLE V. Treatment of chancroid in adults (Based on guidelines from the CDC, from reference 10)

Ceftriaxone 250 mg IM in a single dose+

or

Erythromycin 2.0 gm orally in divided doses for 7 days

or

Sulfamethoxazole-trimethoprim 800/160 mg orally twice daily for 7 days#

+ Avoid for patients with human immunodeficiency virus infection; see text

 # This regimen should be used only if susceptibility of local strains of Haemophilus ducreyi has been documented; 800/160 mg is equivalent to one "double strength" tablet

GENITAL HERPES

Although the clinical picture of genital herpes often is diagnostic, a substantial minority of infections are atypical: many are asymptomatic; others cause minor lesions, the significance of which is not appreciated by the patient or physician; and still others mimic chancroid, syphilis, or other ulcerative conditions.[4,5] Accordingly, attempts should be made to identify HSV by culture or immunochemical methods in all patients with genital ulcers that are not typical of herpes.[4,5] Even for classic cases of genital herpes, the results of culture provide prognostic information that may be useful for some patients. Only a minority of the 10% to 15% of patients whose initial episode of genital herpes is caused by type 1 HSV (HSV-1) will have clinical recurrences, compared with an 80% to 90% rate of recurrence among patients infected with HSV-2.[4] Serological tests are of limited value in diagnosing genital herpes, partly because commercial tests do not accurately distinguish antibody to HSV-2 from that to HSV-1, despite claims to the contrary.[4] Newly developed tests that measure type-specific antibody to HSV glycoprotein G, which are likely to become commercially available in the future, are an important advance, but virus isolation or antigen detection will remain the mainstay of diagnosis.

The clinical classification of genital herpes has an important bearing on treatment and the therapeutic response. *Primary* genital herpes is the patient's first infection with HSV of either type, as evidenced by seronegativity at onset. Most true primary HSV infections apparently are asymptomatic or cause minor nonspecific symptoms, as evidenced by the high prevalence of HSV-2 antibody in sexually active persons who lack histories of genital ulceration.[4] However, clinically apparent primary genital herpes tends to be severe, with large numbers of lesions that may continue to appear over several weeks, regional lymphadenopathy, neuropathic symptoms such as bladder dysfunction or paresthesias in the distribution of the sacral nerve roots, and fever, headache, malaise, or aseptic meningitis.

Recurrent disease is the second or later episode of genital herpes; if type-specific serology is done, antibody to the homologous HSV type is present. Recurrent genital herpes typically is characterized by limited numbers of lesions that are lateralized to one side of the midline, and each recurrence tends to involve the same anatomic region. Regional lymphadenopathy, clinically significant neuropathic manifestations, and systemic symptoms are uncommon.[4]

Non-primary initial genital herpes is the first clinically apparent episode in a person with pre-existing HSV antibody, usually to the opposite HSV type, and all manifestations are midway between recurrent and primary infection in severity and duration.[4]

Acyclovir is the mainstay of therapy for HSV infection. The drug does not eradicate latent infection in the dorsal root ganglia and therefore is not curative,[4] but it is effective in speeding healing of the mucocutaneous lesions. The clinical efficacy of acyclovir is directly correlated with the severity of the clinical episode: the most obvious benefit is observed in true primary disease; less dramatic improvement occurs in initial non-primary HSV infection; and modest or no benefit is observed in most cases of recurrent infection.

Acyclovir should be given IV for primary herpes of sufficient severity to require hospitalization, but outpatient oral therapy is the rule for the large majority of cases. Acyclovir ointment is available, and some patients seem to like the apparently direct approach of applying medication to their lesions, but topical therapy provides little or no objective benefit, and for all stages of infection it is far inferior to systemic therapy.[4] With the exception of treating pregnant women, for whom systemic administration is not approved by the U.S. Food and Drug Administration, the author does not prescribe topical acyclovir.

TABLE VI. Outpatient treatment of genital herpes in adults

Therapeutic Regimen

Acyclovir 200 mg orally five times daily for 5-10 days*

or

Acyclovir 400 mg orally three times daily for 5-10 days*

Prophylactic Regimen

Acyclovir 200 mg orally three times daily+

** Duration of treatment depends on clinical stage and the therapeutic response; see text*

+ May be effective twice daily for some patients; see text.

The outpatient treatment of genital herpes with acyclovir[4,10] is summarized in Table IV. The dosage recommended by the manufacturer for most cases of herpes is 200 mg five times daily (every four hours when awake). However, the plasma half-life of acyclovir is over three hours, and four-hourly administration is based more on the results of the initial clinical studies and habit than on pharmacokinetic factors.[4] The extensive clinical experience of the author and many other authorities indicates that the much more convenient regimen of 400 mg three times daily is equally effective and nontoxic. The bioavailability of orally administered acyclovir is variable, and poor absorption explains some cases of failure of patients to improve within two to three days. In this event, the dose should be doubled to 400 mg five times daily or 800 mg three times daily.[4] These higher doses are recommended routinely for initial episodes of anorectal herpes and for patients with AIDS or other causes of cellular immune deficiency, in whom severe mucocutaneous herpes is common.[4,5]

The usual duration of therapy is ten days for clinically severe episodes (most primary and some initial non-primary cases) and five days to ten days for milder genital herpes in immunologically intact patients. Because acyclovir is expensive, a useful approach is to treat relatively mild cases for five days; if the clinical response is incomplete at the end of this time, the prescription is refilled for five more days. Treatment should always be started as soon as the diagnosis of herpes is suspected, usually prior to virologic confirmation of the diagnosis, because the clinical benefit is largely dependent on early administration.

Most genital herpes recurrences do not benefit from acute treatment with acyclovir; although viral shedding from the lesions is shortened, the time to healing, usually five days to ten days without treatment, is reduced minimally, if at all. On the other hand, very prompt onset of full-dose treatment, at the prodromal stage or immediately upon onset of erythema (before vesiculation occurs), probably provides significant benefit for some patients, sometimes aborting the development of overt lesions.[4] An approach that is practical for some reliable patients who understand their disease and clearly recognize the earliest symptoms is self-administration of a five-day course of acyclovir at the first sign of a recurrence. Prophylactic acyclovir treatment is effective, markedly reducing the frequency of recurrence, with diminished severity and duration of the occasional breakthrough episodes that occur.[4] The usual prophylactic dose is 200 mg three times daily, but twice-daily treatment is effective in some patients. However, the cost and inconvenience of long-term treatment usually make ongoing prophylaxis impractical, except in the unusual patient with especially frequent episodes (e.g., every six weeks or more often) or when the recurrences are very severe or prolonged (e.g., in AIDS patients). Finally, the author occasionally prescribes transient prophylactic therapy, even for patients with infrequent episodes, when avoidance of recurrences is especially important — for example, during a honeymoon or a vacation.

Acyclovir is remarkably nontoxic, causing nausea or headache in $\leq 3\%$ of patients and rarely diarrhea, dizziness, fatigue or other nonspecific symptoms.[4] Because the drug is a purine nucleoside analogue that interferes with replication of viral DNA, there are theoretical concerns about mutagenesis and teratogenicity. Animal studies, however, suggest that such problems are unlikely even at much higher doses than those recommended.[4] Nonetheless, in the absence of clinical data in pregnant women and children, systemic acyclovir is not approved for use for uncomplicated HSV infection in these groups. For the same reason, continuous prophylactic therapy is approved by the U.S. Food and Drug Administration only for a maximal duration of six months, although many patients have taken acyclovir continually for much longer periods without apparent adverse effects. Periodic breaks in prophylactic therapy (every six to twelve months) are suggested to permit reassessment of the frequency and severity of recurrent episodes.[10]

Adjunctive therapy includes keeping the lesions clean with soap and water. Gentle drying of ulcerative lesions with a hair dryer and use of loose-fitting underclothes, perhaps with the addition of cornstarch, may help keep lesions dry and thereby reduce pain, especially when open ulcers are present.[4] Ointments and moisturizing creams (except topical acyclovir) may delay healing. On the other hand, coating of lesions with petroleum jelly or an anesthetic ointment may help some women who have severe dysuria due to urine contacting the lesions; such agents should be washed off after voiding. There is no evidence that any other topical or systemic therapy including vitamins, lysine, other amino acids, or various "immunomodulating" drugs confer any benefit, either in the resolution of acute episodes or in reducing the frequency of recurrences.[4] A few newer chemotherapeutic agents, such as foscarnet (phosphonoformic acid), are under investigation for HSV infection, but so far none appears to have significant advantages over acyclovir.[4]

GENITAL WARTS

Genital warts are caused by any of several types of human papilloma virus (HPV). In the past decade, strong epidemiologic and laboratory data linking some types of HPV (especially types 16 and 18) with squamous cell carcinoma, especially of the cervix, have elevated the perceived importance of this infection from an essentially cosmetic problem to a major public health concern.[6] Visible warts constitute only a small portion of the spectrum of genital HPV infection, and most persons with overt genital lesions also harbor the virus in normal appearing skin or mucosa. In addition, it is likely that many persons with genital HPV infection, perhaps a substantial majority, never develop visible warts yet are infectious for others and are at risk for neoplastic transformation.[6]

The central problem in treatment is that traditional therapies have been intended to ablate overt excrescences (and are inadequate even for this purpose) and are bound to fail to eradicate HPV. Equally important, they are unlikely to completely avert infectivity.[6] Effective therapy for HPV infection in the future will depend on the development of nontoxic systemic chemotherapy or immunotherapy or, alternatively, on much improved local therapy, combined with sensitive methods to identify the presence and anatomic extent of subclinical infection. Although important strides now are being made in identifying persons with subclinical HPV infection, therapeutic refinements have been small and of uncertain clinical application.[15] For practical purposes, eradication of visible warts is all that is available at the present time.

In general, physical ablative methods have been the most effective. Of these, cryotherapy with liquid nitrogen or a cryoprobe is the most effective readily available non-surgical treatment for warts that are not especially extensive.[6,10] Liquid nitrogen is most effectively applied using a spray device, but application by swabs or other devices is an alternative. Visible warts are frozen white, allowed to thaw, then frozen a second time; freeze-thaw cycling seems to enhance efficacy. Two to four treatments at weekly intervals usually are required; the author applies one final treatment after the disappearance of macroscopic lesions. Other physical methods, such as electrocautery, laser therapy, and surgical excision can be effective and require fewer treatments but are less practical for most clinicians. Nevertheless, these methods are the most appropriate for patients with extensive warts, especially when mucosal surfaces are involved. For all physical ablative therapies, the degree of intolerance and "toxicity" depends on the extent of treatment and the depth of tissue destruction; this usually is minimal following cryotherapy and greater following the other methods.[6]

Topical chemotherapy with podophyllin is widely used for genital warts,[6] but probably is less effective than cryotherapy.[15] Podophyllin is a complex, poorly standardized mixture of chemicals extracted from either of two species of the May apple *(Podophyllum sp.)*. It is a potent cellular poison that causes local vasospasm and interferes with cell division by poisoning the mitotic spindle. Not unexpectedly, systemic therapy or excessive local absorption can cause serious toxicity, including death. Podophyllin, usually in an alcoholic solution containing 10% to 25% resin plus benzoin to enhance adherence to treated tissues, is applied directly to the wart, avoiding adjacent skin as much as possible.[6,10] The patient is instructed to wash the material away after two to four hours; with repeated treatments, however, some patients can delay washing for eight and sometimes up to 24 hours without undue local inflammation. Several treatments at weekly intervals usually are required, and visible warts resolve in up to 75% of patients.[6] However, relapse rates of 60% to 80% have been reported in patients followed $\geq$ 3 months after treatment. These rates probably are higher than those following liquid nitrogen cryotherapy,[6] although adequate comparative data are lacking. Virtually all patients develop local erythema, and more severe reactions, including deep ulceration, occasionally occur; the frequency and severity of these reactions can be reduced by avoiding contact of podophyllin with normal skin and washing the material away after a shorter interval.

Fears have been raised about the possibility that podophyllin may be carcinogenic, and most authorities therefore avoid applying it to warts of the uterine cervix.[6,10] Because of the potential for local ulceration and systemic toxicity, most authorities recommend against prescribing podophyllin for self treatment by the patient, preferring to apply it in the office. However, purified podophyllotoxin — one of several active ingredients in podophyllin — has been used experimentally to treat genital warts, with apparently diminished local toxicity, and may be acceptable for self administration.[6] Podophyllin and podophyllotoxin are contraindicated in pregnant women. Topical application of 5-fluorouracil (5-FU) is effective but is used infrequently for external genital warts because of a high frequency of severe and sometimes prolonged local irritation or ulceration.[6] Mucosal warts, however, often respond well to low concentrations of 5-FU, and instillation of a one percent solution is the treatment of choice for intraurethral warts in men. Intravaginal therapy has been used successfully as well. Treatment with 5-FU is contraindicated during pregnancy. Trichloroacetic acid also has been used as ablative therapy for genital warts, but has no clear advantages over other methods.

Various interferons — physiologic immune modulators that also have antiviral characteristics — have been used experimentally for genital warts, both systemically and locally.[15] Systemic therapy to date has had modest efficacy and is limited by toxic effects. Absorption after topical application is low, and in limited studies to date this method has not been very effective. Several studies of intralesional injection have shown promise, but repeated injections are necessary, patient tolerance is poor, and this approach is not clearly superior to cryotherapy or other ablative treatments.[6,15]

CONCLUSION

In summary, the treatment of sexually transmitted diseases has evolved rapidly, due to changes in antimicrobial susceptibility of some pathogens, the development of new antibiotics, and the recognition of the limitations of some formerly recommended regimens. Single dose ceftriaxone, 125 mg to 250 mg intramuscularly (IM), is the initial treatment of choice for gonorrhea. Doxycycline, 100 mg orally twice daily for seven days, is the treatment of choice for uncomplicated chlamydial infection; the same regimen should follow ceftriaxone when heterosexuals are treated for gonorrhea, because many have coexisting chlamydial infection. Various forms of penicillin G remain the mainstay of syphilis therapy. Human immunodeficiency virus (HIV) infection may reduce the responsiveness of central nervous system syphilis to penicillin, and cerebrospinal fluid examination is indicated for all HIV-infected patients with syphilis of any stage. Chancroid is treated either with single dose ceftriaxone, 250 mg, or erythromycin, 2.0 gm daily in divided doses for seven days. Acyclovir has revolutionized the management of genital herpes; oral regimens of 400 mg three times daily or 200 mg five times daily, each for five days to ten days, are highly effective, but topical acyclovir is of little value. No single therapy is uniformly effective for genital warts, partly because subclinical human papilloma virus infection is difficult to identify and treat; cryotherapy with liquid nitrogen or cryoprobe is the treatment of choice for most patients.

REFERENCES

1. Centers for Disease Control. Antibiotic-resistant strains of *Neisseria gonorrhoeae:* policy guidelines for detection, management, and control. MMWR 1988;36(Suppl):1S-18S.
2. Dalabetta G, Hook EW III. Gonococcal infections. Infect Dis Clin North Am 1987;25-4.
3. Stamm WE, Holmes KK. Measures to control *Chlamydia trachomatis* infections: an assessment of new national policy guidelines. JAMA 1986;256:1178-9.
4. Webb DH, Fife KH. Genital herpes simplex virus infections. Infect Dis Clin North Am 1987;1:97-122.
5. Krockta WP, Barnes RC. Genital ulceration with regional lymphadenopathy. Infect Dis Clin North Am 1987;1:217-34.
6. Kirby P, Corey L. Genital human papillomavirus infections. Infect Dis Clin North Am 1987;1:123-44.
7. Handsfield HH. Problems in the treatment of bacterial sexually transmitted diseases. Sex Transm Dis 1986;13(Suppl):179-84.
8. Centers for Disease Control. *Chlamydia trachomatis* infections: policy guidelines for prevention and control. MMWR 1985;34 (Suppl):53S-74S.

9. Batteiger BE, Jones RB. *Chlamydia* infections. Infect Dis Clin North Am 1987;1:55-82.
10. Centers for Disease Control. Sexually transmitted diseases treatment guidelines, 1989. MMWR (in press).
11. Handsfield HH, Hook EW III. Ceftriaxone for treatment of uncomplicated gonorrhea: routine use in a sexually transmitted disease clinic. Sex Transm Dis 1987;14:226-30.
12. Lukehart SA. Current issues in syphilis therapy. STD Bulletin 1988;8(2):2-15.
13. Lukehart SA, Hook EW III, Baker-Zander SA, et al. Invasion of the central nervous system by *Treponema pallidum:* implications for diagnosis and therapy. Ann Intern Med 1988;109:855-62.
14. Hooton TM, Barnes RC. Urethritis in men. Infect Dis Clin North Am 1987;1:165-78.
15. Kirby P. Interferon and genital warts. JAMA 1988;259:570-2.

CHAPTER 4

Outpatient Management of Gynecologic Infections

Alan Berkeley, M.D.
New York, New York

INTRODUCTION

Current medical practice stresses preventive care, early diagnosis, and outpatient therapies at the lowest possible cost. Many female genital infections have traditionally been treated as outpatient conditions. There is, however, a growing recognition that many vaginal, cervical and upper genital tract diseases represent a continuum. While outpatient therapy may be appropriate, the serious sequelae from untreated forms of these diseases may ultimately lead to higher health care costs in general. It is therefore important for the practitioner to have an organized approach to the diagnosis and treatment of gynecologic infections. In this way, those infections that are minor, although bothersome, can be separated from those that have more serious implications. This review will focus on the management of vaginitis, cervicitis, and pelvic inflammatory disease (PID) in the outpatient setting.

VAGINITIS

The treatment of vaginitis has been a challenge to gynecologists for many years. Osborne demonstrated that a cohort of college students presenting with symptoms of vulvovaginitis, as compared with a group of asymptomatic women, had statistically significantly higher isolation rates for *Trichomonas, Candida, Gardnerella,* herpes simplex, gonococci, and *Chlamydia*.[1] The gynecologist must therefore recognize the differences among these various infectious agents, both in terms of symptoms, and in terms of implications for more serious upper genital tract disease.

Etiology

Approximately one quarter of vaginitis cases are caused by yeast organisms, about 85% of which are *Candida albicans*.[2,3] Another 10% are caused by *Torulopsis glabrata*,[4] and the remaining cases are probably caused by *Candida tropicalis*.[5] Colonization rates in normal asymptomatic patients have been reported as being anywhere from 10% to 55%.[1,3]

Yeast Infection

About 75% of adult women will have at least one symptomatic attack of yeast vaginitis during their lifetime. The *Candida* organism has both a yeast and a pseudohyphae form. Pseudohyphae formation enhances adherence to and invasion of mucosal tissues.

Although many risk factors have been identified with the development of yeast vaginitis, many cases occur in patients with no recognized risk factors. Those factors that appear to be associated with the development of this condition include the usage of broad spectrum antibiotics, pregnancy, diabetes mellitus, and an immunosuppressed state. Although some investigators have found an increase in yeast colonization in women using oral contraceptives, the actual incidence of symptomatic yeast infections in these patients does not appear to be different than that in patients not using oral contraception.[3] It has also often been suggested that the use of tight-fitting clothing such as blue jeans or the wearing of silk underwear promotes yeast infections. Uncircumcised male partners may also represent a source for yeast; however, the role of sexual transmittal is unclear since 80% of male partners of women with yeast infections are culture negative for the organism, and, in addition, many women who have yeast infections are celibate.

In cases of vaginitis, patients present with a cheesy, white vaginal discharge that is often adherent to the vaginal walls. The vaginal and vulvar tissues may be edematous and reddened. The patient may complain of severe internal and/or external pruritus, and there is often marked dyspareunia. The diagnosis is usually made by means of a 10% potassium hydroxide wet-mount in which the classic yeast or pseudohyphae forms can be seen. It is rarely necessary to culture on Sabouraud's medium. Vaginal pH is usually between 4.5 and 5, and the number of white cells in the vaginal smear is usually not increased.

FIGURE 1. Risk factors for yeast vulvovaginitis

1) Broad spectrum antibiotics
2) Pregnancy
3) Diabetes Mellitus
4) Immunosuppression
5) ? Oral contraception
6) ? Increased genital temperature and humidity (blue jeans, silk underwear)
7) ? Uncircumcized male consort

Therapy for Isolated Attacks

Treatment of yeast vulvovaginitis usually falls into one of two categories, depending on whether the case is an isolated attack or a recurrent infection. The isolated attack usually responds to topical therapy with either cream or suppositories. The traditional polyene antifungal agent, nystatin, has for the most part been replaced by the imidazole derivatives, miconazole and clotrimazole.

These latter have the advantage of both shorter duration of therapy (usually three to seven days) and somewhat higher cure rates with one treatment (usually in the range of 80% to 90%).[6,7,8] Newer agents such as ketoconazole (oral and topical) and terconazole (topical) also have high single treatment success rates.[9] Topical treatment with 1% gentian violet has also been advocated for resistant cases, although this can be quite messy and irritating if used continuously.

Therapy for Chronic Recurrent Infections

The patient with chronic recurrent yeast infections represents a much more difficult treatment problem. The infections almost always represent a persistence of the same organism rather than a completely new infection, since retreatment with the same agent often works.[7,10] This repeated infection may be from genital seeding from a gastrointestinal source,[11] from re-exposure to an infected sexual contact, or from the presence of several of the more accepted risk factors, particularly pregnancy and compromised immunity. Any attempt to eradicate these infections must also treat these predisposing conditions, if present. These patients may require chronic suppression, but the infection often recurs once suppression is terminated.

Witkin and Ledger[12] have shown that some cases of recurrent yeast vaginitis may represent "immunologic vaginitis." Peripheral lymphocyte proliferation is reduced or absent in three-quarters of patients with recurrent *Candida* infections and sera from these patients can also inhibit lymphocyte proliferation. These reactions are prostaglandin-mediated and can be lessened by anti-prostaglandins, such as ibuprofen. In addition, vaginal wash specimens that contain yeast filaments or anti-*Candida* IgE are associated with recurrent disease. Finally, other studies[12] have shown a role for histamine-mediated reactions, and treatment with certain antihistamines may offer some hope to this subgroup of patients.

FIGURE 2. Yeast vulvovaginitis treatment alternatives

1) Nystatin suppositories (100,000 units) or cream bid X 14 days
2) Miconazole cream 2% (Monistat) qhs X 7 days
3) Clotriamazole suppositories (100 mg) or cream (Gyne-Lotrimin) qhs X 3 or 7 days
4) Tetconazole suppositories (80 mg) or 0.4% cream (Terazol) qhs X 3 or 7 days
5) Gentian Violet 1% topically twice weekly
6) Nystatin Tablets (100,000 units) orally bid (No systemic absorption)
7) Ketoconazole Tablets (200 mg) orally qd (systemic absorption)

Trichomonal Infections

Trichomonas vaginitis represents approximately one-quarter of the cases of vaginitis.[2] This sexually transmitted motile protozoan can be carried by its human host asymptomatically, but usually causes a copious yellow-green, sometimes frothy, vaginal discharge and marked vaginal burning and pruritus. The discharge is malodorous.

Many investigators have described a strawberry cervix with many patchy red areas that can also be seen on colposcopic exam. This finding, however, is not diagnostic and often not present. The diagnosis is usually made on a wet-mount where the motile protozoan can be seen. The chance of a wet-mount being positive is directly related to the concentration of the *Trichomonas* in the vaginal secretions. The higher the concentration, the more likely the wet mount is to be positive. Culture in Diamonds media is rarely necessary unless there are recurrent infections and a suggestion of antibiotic resistance.

Metronidazole has been the mainstay of therapy for trichomonal infection. A single, two gram dose for the patient and her consort, given simultaneously, will cure about 90% of the patients and will usually have a higher compliance rate than the more traditional 250 mg three times daily, for one week treatment. The patient should be warned not to drink alcohol during the course of the treatment because of a possible disulfiram-type reaction. Metronidazole is usually well tolerated, with gastrointestinal discomfort being the most common side effect. The patient should have a follow-up exam shortly after treatment to confirm eradication of the organism. While there has been some concern about the carcinogenic potential of metronidazole, because of data from animal models,[13,14] there has not been evidence for any increase in human cancer or congenital anomalies after pregnancy exposure.[15] However, it is a good idea to confirm that the patient is neither pregnant nor at risk for pregnancy before initiating treatment with metronidazole.

There are rare cases of trichomonal resistance to metronidazole. These patients can usually be cured by high dose inpatient intravenous therapy with metronidazole, which is often combined with vaginal metronidazole.

Bacterial Vaginosis

Bacterial vaginosis (BV) is the designation given to what was formerly categorized as non-specific vaginitis, *Gardnerella* vaginitis, or *Hemophilus* vaginitis.

Diagnosis

Thomason[16,17] has suggested that the clinical diagnosis can be made if four of the five following criteria are met: (1) there is a gray, homogeneous vaginal discharge that often coats the external genitalia and is associated with burning and pruritus, although vulvovaginal irritation is not a prominent feature; (2) the vaginal pH is usually between 5 and 5.5; (3) a fishy, amine odor can be elicited by adding KOH to a vaginal sample; (4) a wet-mount reveals the presence of "clue cells," which are epithelial cells laden with small gram-negative bacteria to such a degree that their margins become indistinct; and, (5) a wet-mount shows an increase in density of small background bacteria accompanied by a decrease in normal lactobacilli morphotypes.

Etiology

BV is associated with between a 100 and 1000 time increase in the vaginal colonization with anaerobic organisms, particularly *Bacteroides* and the more recently identified *Mobiluncus*. Increased organic acid from anaerobes and vaginal secretions can be detected by gas/liquid chromatography. Most investigators believe that a succinic acid to lactic acid ratio of greater than 0.4 is positive for the presence of bacterial vaginosis, since succinate is produced by *Mobiluncus* and *Gardnerella*, but not by lactobacilli.[18] In addition, a variety of organisms, including those associated with bacterial vaginosis, are reported to produce prolineaminopeptidase, and testing for this enzyme will identify approximately 80% of cases.[19] Indirectly, the prominent role played by an overgrowth of anaerobic bacteria is demonstrated by the clinical response of this condition to metronidazole, an antimicrobial highly effective against anaerobic bacteria.

Hillier[20] has demonstrated the protective role of lactobacilli, particularly those which produce hydrogen peroxide, a compound toxic to bacteria that do not produce catalase. The presence in the vagina of peroxide-producing lactobacilli should inhibit the growth of the anaerobic bacteria associated with bacterial vaginosis. This inhibitory effect can be overcome by any condition that causes a higher vaginal pH or a larger inoculum of bacteria. Two such events might be menses or intercourse.

Sequelae

There is growing evidence that the presence of BV predisposes a woman to a more serious spectrum of bacterial infections. These associations include preterm labor, preterm rupture of membranes, amniotic fluid injection, and pelvic inflammatory disease.[21,22,23] If these associations do exist, the mandate for treating all cases of bacterial vaginosis would become that much more compelling. It has been suggested that the presence of BV increases the likelihood of post-operative infections from gynecologic procedures, and Watts has suggested repeatedly[24] that the presence of these organisms increases the risk for postpartum endometritis, despite antibiotic prophylaxis.

Treatment

The treatment of bacterial vaginosis is metronidazole 500 mg orally twice daily for one week.[25] During pregnancy, amoxicillin 500 mg, four times daily for one week will provide some relief of symptoms but is considerably less effective than metronidazole. The topical vaginal use of yogurt-based lactobacillus, estrogen cream, or acetic acid jelly has not been as effective as metronidazole.[26] There is no evidence that the treatment of sexual partners increases the efficacy of treatment, although many experts treat the partner when infection recurs. It is often helpful to have the couple use condoms until the infection clears.

Carmona[27] has published a non-comparative study of oral ciprofloxacin 500 mg bid for seven days in 22 women suffering from nonspecific vaginitis which had been present for one to three months. Clinical and bacteriologic responses were evaluated seven days after the last day of ciprofloxacin treatment. Seventeen of the 22 enrolled (77.3%) were cured, four (18.2%) showed improvement and only one (4.5%) showed clinical failure. Overall, eighteen (81.8%) had a successful bacteriologic response. Side effects consisted of mild to moderate gastric pain, dizziness, somnolence and pruritus. In no case did ciprofloxacin therapy have to be discontinued because of side effects.

PELVIC INFLAMMATORY DISEASE (PID)

If a patient presents with pain, as well as with vaginal discharge, it is important to make the differential diagnosis between early pelvic inflammatory disease (PID) and vaginitis. Brunham[28] has described a syndrome called mucopurulent endocervicitis that is associated with *Chlamydia trachomatis* in about 50% of cases. The hallmark of this condition is a highly inflamed cervix with mucopus in the endocervical secretions. Women with this condition are much more likely to have *Chlamydia* isolated from endometrium, and, therefore, this vaginal discharge really represents an initial stage of PID.

Seriousness of PID

There is a tendency to consider diseases treated in an outpatient setting as being less serious than those that require hospitalization. Although there may be several stages of PID that can be adequately treated as an outpatient, it is important for the physician to bear in mind the extremely serious sequelae this disease can have for the patient. Although there are nearly one million cases per year of gonorrhea, approximately four million new cases per year of *Chlamydia*, and approximately one million symptomatic episodes of PID, only about 25% of the symptomatic patients will be hospitalized for treatment. The sequelae of PID include infertility, ectopic pregnancy, chronic pelvic pain, and recurrent episodes of pelvic infection. The goal of treatment should therefore be not only alleviation of symptoms, but also prevention of gross injuries to pelvic structures.

Data from Westrum in Scandinavia[29] make it clear that after one symptomatic attack of pelvic infection approximately 11% of patients will suffer tubal occlusion. This incidence increases to 23% after two attacks, and approximately 50% after three attacks. Even more patients will suffer lesser degrees of tubal damage that compromise fertility.

Over the last twenty years there has been approximately a tripling of the incidence of ectopic pregnancy. Part of this increase may be due to more sensitive pregnancy tests and increased use of tubal reconstructive surgery. At least half of this increase has been attributed to an increasing incidence of sexually transmitted PID. Since approximately 12% of maternal mortality in this country is related to ectopic pregnancy, approximately 6% of maternal mortality, or about 900 deaths per year, can be attributed to pelvic infection.

FIGURE 3. Sequelae of Pelvic Inflammatory Disease

1) Infertility
2) Ectopic pregnancy (of those who become pregnant after PID, 5% will have ectopic gestation)
3) Chronic pelvic pain in 20%
4) Recurrent PID in approximately 25%

Risk Factors for PID

Risk factors for PID can be generalized into four categories. The most important factor is the number of sexual partners, with an increasing risk for infection with more partners. The second major factor is the sexual history of the male partner. Prior practice was to involve the male partner in the evaluation of pelvic infection only if gonorrhea was isolated. Contemporary practice mandates that the male be involved in the treatment of pelvic infection in every case of female pelvic infection. The third factor relating to the incidence of PID is the type of contraception used, with those using an intrauterine device more at risk. Finally, the general health or socio-economic background of a given patient will determine her ability to withstand infection.

It should be noted that most men with bacteriospermia are asymptomatic, and that the severity of bacteriospermia is often related to the number of prior sexual partners.[30] Women who are married to men with higher bacterial counts in their seminal fluid are more likely to develop PID, since the bacterial component of seminal fluid is added to the cervical and vaginal flora during intercourse.

Toth[31] has shown that, in the presence of sperm, aerobic and anaerobic bacteria can migrate through ovulatory phase cervical mucous; however this migration did not occur in the absence of sperm. Indirect proof of this finding is the fact that the wives of men who are aspermic rarely develop PID.[31] Interestingly, this migration did not occur when mucous from the luteal phase or pregnancy was used. It may be that the frequent clinical observation that initiation of an episode of pelvic inflammation occurs at the time of menses is related to loss of protection from cervical mucous.

Although the use of intrauterine contraceptive devices for birth control has decreased markedly over the last ten years, some IUDs are still on the market, and many patients still have their IUDs in place. Although many of the epidemiologic studies performed were flawed by the fact that control groups contained patients who were at less than average risk for the development of PID (such as birth control pill users), most studies documented a several-fold increased relative risk of pelvic infection in the presence of an IUD.[32,33,34] The effect of IUDs to increase the risk for PID was most dramatic in the instance of Dalkon Shield users and was least marked for those who used copper-containing devices. The mechanisms of this increased risk include the tail of the IUD acting as a conduit for bacteria, trauma to the endometrium from the IUD itself, increasing access of bacteria to the endometrial cavity, and the menorrhagia often caused by IUDs acting as an excellent culture media. Dahling[35] has also shown that the incidence of primary tubal infertility is directly related to prior usage of an IUD, with the risk being highest for Dalkon Shield users and lowest for copper-bearing IUD users.

Bacteriologic Etiology of PID

Over the last five to ten years, a better understanding has developed of the bacteriology of many of the infections causing PID. It has been learned that there is often a tremendous difference in the presenting signs and symptoms, depending on the causative organism.[36] Gonococcal PID often presents as acute illness with duration of symptoms for less than 24 hours. On the other hand, chlamydial PID often presents a more indolent infection that has been present for longer than 48 hours with less acute symptoms.[37]

It is unlikely that any physician would fail to recognize an acute case of gonococcal salpingitis; however, not all asymptomatic carriers of gonorrhea will progress to upper genital tract disease, and, unfortunately, many patients with asymptomatic lower genital tract disease will not be recognized until they present in an acute condition. In a study of reasons for failure to identify cases of asymptomatic gonorrhea, Platt[38] has pointed out that many STD clinics do not perform bimanual exams or tests for gonorrhea routinely, even in patients with pelvic complaints. Many patients with minimal symptomatology are never thoroughly evaluated; thus there is a long delay in their definitive treatment. It is imperative that every patient with pelvic symptomatology or vaginal discharge be evaluated for the presence of sexually transmitted organisms. Those women at high risk as defined by sexual practice, socio economic status, or known infected male partner, should also be thoroughly evaluated.

ROLE OF CHLAMYDIA

The role of *Chlamydia trachomatis* in pelvic infection is now clearly recognized. At least 50% of cases of non-specific urethritis in males and mucopurulent endocervicitis in females is of chlamydial etiology.[28] At least half of patients with chlamydial carriage will have no symptoms; and those who have infection will often not have a painful course, a fever, or an elevated white count and, therefore, may delay in seeking medical attention.[37]

Although *Chlamydia* was isolated from one-quarter to one-third of endocervical and intraperitoneal cultures in Scandinavia,[39,40] these findings were not initially corroborated in the United States.[41,42] With the recognition that *Chlamydia* is an obligative intracellular parasite came the understanding that viable cellular material was required in order to get a positive culture. The evidence for chlamydial involvement in PID includes the following: increased positive cervical and intraperitoneal cultures in PID patients as compared with control subjects; positive IgG microimmunofluorescence greater than 1:64 more frequently found in PID patients as compared with control subjects (62% vs 11%); and the fact that more infertile patients than pregnant control subjects have antibodies to *Chlamydia*. This difference in antibody titer between PID patients and control subjects is even more dramatic when those patients with tubal occlusion on hysterosalpingogram are compared with those with patent tubes. Henry-Suchet showed a statistically increased isolation of *Chlamydia* from both the cervix and the peritoneum in patients with acute PID, infertility, or both, as compared to a fertile control group.[43] There was also a marked increase in positivity of serology in these patients.

The importance of *Chlamydia* is not limited to pelvic infection and its sequelae of infertility and ectopic pregnancy.[44] There is an effect on the children born to women with *Chlamydia* colonization at the time of delivery; approximately 20% of such neonates will develop chlamydial conjunctivitis, and approximately 15% of such neonates will develop chlamydial pneumonia. It is also suspected that women colonized with *Chlamydia* have an increased incidence of premature rupture of membranes and pre-term delivery,[21] which appears particularly true for women with positive IgM serology suggestive of upper genital tract disease or more recent infection.[45]

Laboratory Detection of Chlamydia

The identification of *Chlamydia* has been complicated because of its life cycle. Over approximately a 48-hour time span, the extracellular form of this organism, the elementary body, is phagocytosed by a cell inside which it multiplies into the intracellular form, the reticulate body. These bodies multiply until cell lysis occurs. This predominantly intracellular life cycle has particular importance for successful isolation of *Chlamydia*. Material obtained from the cul-de-sac often has little cellular debris or viable cellular tissue, and rarely will a positive culture turn up from this material. Material for culture should be obtained by calcium alginate swabs and plated out on McCoy's cell culture. *Chlamydia* can be recognized by Giesma staining or monoclonal antibody staining of the intracellular bodies. Both monoclonal and ELISA direct staining methods of cellular material are now available; their only drawback is an approximate 2% false positivity rate, which is important in low prevalence populations, where a significant percent of positive tests will represent false positives. Therefore, where the prevalence is low, identification by culture, rather than by immunology may still be required for definitive diagnosis.

Further suggestive evidence for the role of *Chlamydia* in these infections is the finding that women with ectopic pregnancies will have a markedly increased isolation of *Chlamydia* antibodies as compared with a control group.[46]

Diagnosis of PID

The diagnosis of PID is often difficult. Hager's criteria[47] for the diagnosis include lower abdominal pain with cervical motion tenderness and adnexal tenderness, as well as at least one of the following: temperature greater than 38°C, leukocytosis, culdocentesis with fluid containing white blood cells and bacteria, an elevated sedimentation rate, a Gram's stain of the cervical smear containing gram-negative intracellular gram-negative diplococci, or a monoclonal smear of endocervical secretions revealing *Chlamydia.* If available, ultrasonic confirmation of an inflammatory pelvic mass would also help in the diagnosis. However, there is tremendous overlap between patients who are laparoscopically proven to have salpingitis and those who are laparoscopically proven not to have salpingitis, in terms of almost all the signs and symptoms commonly used to make this diagnosis. Jacobson[48] demonstrated that in only about 65% of cases will laparoscopy confirm the diagnosis of pelvic infection, with nearly a quarter of the patients having a normal pelvis at the time of operation. In addition, a significant number of patients will be admitted to a hospital with other diagnoses that ultimately prove to be PID. It is, therefore, important to utilize laparoscopy in those cases where the diagnosis is in doubt or where the clinical response to antibiotic therapy has been minimal or absent.

It is also important to obtain adequate material for microbiologic evaluation. The polymicrobial etiology of salpingitis has been recognized for some time, but cultures obtained from the endocervix or via culdocentesis will often reveal lower genital tract contaminants rather than upper genital tract pathogens.[49] Therefore, one should obtain endometrial cultures via triple lumen catheters or intraperitoneal cultures via laparoscopy.

FIGURE 4. Criteria for admission for acute PID

1) Diagnosis is uncertain (appendicitis and ectopic pregnancy must be excluded)
2) Presence of pelvic abscess or inflammatory adnexal mass
3) Severe abdominal pain, including rebound tenderness
4) Temperature > 38° C
5) Gastrointestinal symptoms preclude oral medications
6) Pregnancy
7) Presence of intrauterine device
8) Failure to respond to outpatient therapy
9) Clinical follow-up cannot be arranged

Ambulatory Therapy vs Hospitalization for PID

Despite the tremendous impact of these infections on rates of infertility and ectopic pregnancy, no definitive data exists concerning whether inpatient or outpatient therapy is more efficacious in preventing sequelae. Because of the seriousness of the possible complications, it is tempting to admit all women with symptomatic PID for inpatient therapy. However, at the present time nearly three-quarters of symptomatic cases are not admitted.[50] Because of the potential cost and manpower inpact of these additional admissions on the health care system of the U.S., it appears logistically and economically unfeasible to admit all patients with symptomatic PID.

Patients who are candidates for admission, and for whom outpatient therapy would probably be inappropriate, include:[51] (1) those who have a fever greater than 38°C; (2) those with significant pelvic or upper abdominal pain, including rebound tenderness; (3) those whose gastrointestinal symptoms preclude the effective use of oral medications; (4) those who have an intrauterine device *in situ*; (5) those who are pregnant; (6) those who have inflammatory adnexal masses; (7) those who fail to respond to 48 hours of outpatient therapy or who worsen on outpatient therapy; and (8) those whose diagnosis is in doubt (suspected appendicitis or ectopic pregnancy).

In my experience many patients who fulfill some of these criteria are still being treated as outpatients, but probably every effort should be made to admit them.

Once a decision has been made to treat PID on an outpatient basis, treatment strategies must include antimicrobial therapies directed at gonorrhea, *Chlamydia* and anaerobic organisms.[52] In fact, it is no longer acceptable to treat only for gonorrhea, as was documented by Stamm.[53] He compared three traditional protocols: (1) intramuscular penicillin plus probenecid; (2) nine tablets daily of trimethoprim/sulfamethoxazole daily for three days; or (3) tetracycline 500 mg qid for five days. An important finding was the failure of the tetracycline protocol to eradicate gonorrhea in 10% of his patients. Conversely, those patients treated only with penicillin had less than a 50% eradication rate of *Chlamydia* and a higher incidence of post-gonococcal urethritis and cervicitis. Also, salpingitis developed significantly more frequently in those treated only with penicillin.

Of note, Washington[54] has demonstrated the cost-effectiveness of a combined approach. His data reveal that treatment directed against both *Chlamydia* and gonorrhea, using two antibiotics, will be more efficacious than therapy directed against only one of these agents. Based on inpatient data, Sweet[55] has also demonstrated that treatment of PID with a cephalosporin only, without coverage for *Chlamydia*, results in incomplete eradication of *Chlamydia* from the endometrium. Although these patients were clinically cured, the failure to eradicate *Chlamydia* provides a possible explanation for relapse or chronic tubal infection. In addition, Center for Disease Control (CDC) protocols for inpatient therapy all include antibiotics that treat both gonorrhea and *Chlamydia*.[52]

FIGURE 5. Treatment of uncomplicated gonorrhea

1) Acqueous Procaine Penicillin G 4.8 million units IM at 2 sites with Probenecid 1 gm orally
2) Amoxicillin 3 gm or Ampicillin 3.5 gm orally with 1 gm Probenecid
3) Ceftriaxone 250 mg IM or Cefoxitin 2 gm IM with 1 gm Probenecid
4) Spectinomycin 2 gm IM (in case of penicillin allergy)
5) Erythromycin 1.5 gm orally followed by 500 mg qid for seven days (for pregnant patients with penicillin allergy)

All to be followed by either:
1) Doxycycline 100 mg bid orally X 7 days or
2) Tetracycline 500 mg qid orally X 7 days

Penicillin-Resistant Gonorrhea

Further complicating outpatient therapy is the emergence of penicillinase-producing gonorrhea. In most urban areas, the incidence of these penicillin-resistant strains of gonorrhea approaches 2%.[56] Therefore, in such urban areas it is no longer appropriate to treat gonorrhea with intramuscular penicillin. Conversely, in those areas with a low prevalence of resistant organisms (< 1 %), it is probably still appropriate to use 4.8 million units of intramuscular procaine penicillin with one gram of probenecid, as long as the patient will be available for "test-of-cure" cultures following treatment, including susceptibility testing.[57]

Where there is a high incidence of penicillin-resistant strains of gonorrhea, the usually recommended intramuscular therapy is 250 mg of ceftriaxone, or one or two grams of cefoxitin. However, since evidence of gonorrhea resistance to cefoxitin has been reported,[58] ceftriaxone 250 mg intramuscularly is the antibiotic of choice. In patients allergic to penicillin or cephalosporin antibiotics, spectinomycin 2 gm intramuscularly would also be appropriate therapy. The important point to stress is that all of these intramuscular dosages must be followed by either doxycycline 100 mg twice daily for seven days or tetracycline 500 mg four times daily for seven days. I personally prefer doxycycline because of better patient compliance with fewer dosages, as well as slightly better anaerobic coverage.

Pregnant patients who are not candidates for treatment with doxycycline or metronidazole can be treated with erythromycin 500 mg four times daily for seven days, although this can lead to troublesome gastrointestinal side effects that require lowering the dose to 250 mg, four times daily for 14 days.[59]

More Recent Therapies of PID

While the traditional regimens for treatment of PID require treatment with two antibiotics, some of the new quinolone antimicrobials may allow treatment for both gonorrhea and *Chlamydia* with a single antibiotic agent.[60] Our experience with ofloxacin 400 mg twice daily for ten days showed clinical cure in 17 of 18 patients. All isolates of *Chlamydia* and gonorrhea were eradicated. These results compared favorably to parallel randomized treatment with cefoxitin 2 gm intramuscularly followed by ten days of doxycycline. Many more patients will need to be evaluated to determine whether this initially good experience will become an acceptable outpatient therapy.

Importance of Follow-Up Therapy

Finally, one cannot stress strongly enough the importance of rapid and definitive follow-up in women treated as outpatients for salpingitis or endometritis. Our experience has been that those patients with acute onset illness are rapidly cured by almost any combination of antibiotics and rarely require either surgical intervention or changing of antibiotic therapy. On the other hand, those patients with established infections that have been allowed to simmer over days or weeks have a much poorer outcome; they have a higher incidence of inflammatory adnexal masses and surgical intervention, and there is usually a requirement for multiple antibiotic therapy. Patients should be instructed that if symptoms become worse, they should call the treating physican or return to the treatment facility immediately for additional care. In addition, patients should be given appointments for follow-up examination 48 hours following initiation of therapy. Failure of a patient to respond to treatment mandates admission and further evaluation, a situation that is particularly important in a clinic setting, where follow-up is often sub-optimal.

Consort Therapy

It is now our policy to treat the male partner of every female patient who is diagnosed as having PID. If gonorrhea is isolated, this includes combination therapy directed at both the gonococcus and the *Chlamydia*. It is well documented that approximately one-quarter of patients with gonorrhea will also have *Chlamydia* isolated. Even in the absence of gonococcal isolation, the male partner is treated with doxycycline twice daily for seven to ten days.

Outpatient Therapy Following Hospitalization

It has been common practice for patients to be treated with one of the various CDC inpatient protocols[52] until they have been afebrile and asymptomatic for 48 to 72 hours. At that point patients have traditionally been discharged on doxycycline for an additional seven to ten days to complete treatment of *Chlamydia*. Some attending physicians, in addition, treat with either clindamycin or metronidazole to eradicate the anaerobic organisms that are presumed to be involved in these polymicrobial infections. Of interest is a recent report by Hager,[61] who prospectively and randomly treated half of his discharged patients with antibiotics and half without. He could identify no difference in any outcome variable, including the need for subsequent readmission. In those patients without inflammatory adnexal masses, it is possible that inpatient therapy that includes coverage for *Chlamydia* is all that is required for effective resolution of symptoms.

CONCLUSION

The spectrum of female genital infections runs the gamut from the asymptomatic colonization with organisms that have no long-term prognostic significance to those infections that are acutely uncomfortable or painful with dire implications for future fertility and reproductive health. It is the responsibility of the practicing physician to make a correct diagnosis, institute appropriate treatment, and provide adequate follow-up care. If discovered and treated early in their course, virtually all of these infections are amenable to outpatient therapy, with minimal or no compromise of reproductive health.

REFERENCES

1. Osborne NG, Grubin L, Pratson L. Vaginitis in sexually active women: relationship to nine sexually transmitted organisms. Am J Obstet Gynecol 1982;142:962-7.
2. Gardner H, Dukes CD. *Haemophilus vaginalis* vaginitis: a newly defined specific infection previously classified "nonspecific" vaginitis. Am J Obstet Gynecol 1955;69:962-76.
3. Oriel JD, Partridge BM, Denny MJ, et al. Genital yeast infections. Br Med J 1972;4:761-4.

4. Smith AG, Taubert HD, Martin CW. The use of trichomycin in the treatment of vulvovaginal mycosis in pregnant women. Am J Obstet Gynecol 1963;87:455-62.
5. Nagesha CN, Ananthakrishna NC. Clinical and laboratory study of monilial vaginitis. Am J Obstet Gynecol 1970;107:1267-8.
6. Davis JE, Frudenfeld JH, Goddard JL. Comparative evaluation of monistat and mycostatin in the treatment of vulvovaginal candidiasis. Obstet Gynecol 1974;44:403-6.
7. McNellis D, McLeod M, Lawson J, et al. Treatment of vulvovaginal candidiasis in pregnancy: a comparative study. Obstet Gynecol 1977;50:674-8.
8. Tan CG, Milne LJR, Good CS, et al. A comparative trial of six-day therapy with clotrimazole and nystatin in pregnant patients with vaginal candidiasis. Postgrad Med J 1974; 50:Suppl 1:102.
9. Heel RC, Brogden RN, Carmine A, et al. Ketoconazole: a review of its therapeutic efficacy in superficial and systemic fungal infections. Drugs 1982;23:1-36.
10. Van Syke KK, Michel VP, Rein MF. Treatment of vulvovaginal candidiasis with boric acid powder. Am J Obstet Gynecol 1981; 141:145-98.
11. Miles MR, Olsen L, Rogers A. Recurrent vaginal candidiasis. Importance of an intestinal reservoir. JAMA 1977;238:1836-7.
12. Witkin SS, Ledger WJ. Association between eosinophils in vaginal smears and vaginal allergic responses in women with recurrent vaginitis. Infect Dis Soc Obstet Gynecol 1988. abstract.
13. Rustia M, Shubik P. Induction of lung tumors and malignant lymphomas in mice by metronidazole. J Nat Cancer Inst 1972; 48:721-6.
14. Legator MS, Connor TH, Stoeckel M. Detection of mutagenic activity of metronidazole and niridazole in body fluids of humans and mice. Science 1975;188:1118-9.
15. Morgan I. Metronidazole treatment in pregnancy. Int J Gynaecol Obstet 1978;15:501-2.
16. Thomason JL, Schreckenberger PC, Spellacy WN. Clinical and microbiological characterization of patients with nonspecific vaginosis associated with motile, curved anaerobic rods. J Infect Dis 1984;149:801-9.
17. Mead PB, Thomason JL, Ledger WJ, et al. Establishing bacterial vaginosis. Contemp Obstet Gynecol 1986;27:89.
18. Ison CA, Easmon CS, Dawson SG, et al. Non-volatile fatty acids in the diagnosis of non-specific vaginitis. J Clin Pathol 1983;36:1367-70.
19. Thomason JL, Gelbart SM, Wilcoski LM, et al. Prolineaminopeptidase activity as a rapid diagnostic test to confirm bacterial vaginosis. Obstet Gynecol 1988;71:607-11.
20. Hillier SL. *In vitro* inhibition of vaginal microorganisms by lactobacilli. Infect Dis Soc Obstet Gynecol 1988. abstract.
21. Gravett MG, Nelson HP, DeRouen T, et al. Independent associations of bacterial vaginosis and *Chlamydia trachomatis* infection with adverse pregnancy outcome. JAMA 1986;256:1899-903.
22. Gravett MG, Hummel D, Eschenbach DA, et al. Preterm labor associated with subclinical amniotic fluid infection and with bacterial vaginosis. Obstet Gynecol 1986;67:229-37.
23. Eschenbach DA, Hillier SL, Critchlow C, et al. Diagnosis and clinical manifestations of bacterial vaginosis. Am J Obstet Gynecol 1988;158:819-28.
24. Watts DH, Krohn MA, Hillier SL, et al. Abnormal vaginal flora as a risk factor for postcesarean section endometritis. Infect Dis Soc Obstet Gynecol 1988. abstract.
25. Pheifer TA, Forsyth PS, Durfee MA, et al. Non-specific vaginitis: role of *Haemophilus vaginalis* and treatment with metronidazole. N Engl J Med 1978;298:1429-34.
26. Fredricsson B, Englund K, Weintraub L, et al. Ecological treatment of bacterial vaginosis. Lancet 1987;(letter)(8527):276.
27. Carmona O, Silva H, Acosta H, et al. Tinidazol en al tratamiento de vaginitis inespecifiacas asociada a *Gardnerella vaginalis* y bacterias anaerobicas. Investigacion

Medica Internacional 1983;10:Suppl 3:23.
28. Brunham RC, Paavonen J, Stevens CE, et al. Mucopurulent cervicitis — the ignored counterpart in women of urethritis in men. N Engl J Med 1984;311:1-6.
29. Westtrom L. Incidence, prevalence, and trends of acute pelvic inflammatory disease and its consequences in industrialized countries. Am J Obstet Gynecol 1980;138:880-92.
30. Toth A, Lesser ML. Asymptomatic bacteriospermia in fertile and infertile men. Fertil Steril 1981;36:88-91.
31. Toth A, O'Leary WM, Ledger W. Evidence for microbial transfer by spermatozoa. Obstet Gynecol 1982;59:556-9.
32. Eschenbach DA, Harnisch JP, Holmes KK. Pathogenesis of acute pelvic inflammatory disease: role of contraception and other risk factors. Am J Obstet Gynecol 1977;128:838-50.
33. Westrom L, Bengtsson L, Mardh P-A. The risk of pelvic inflammatory disease in women using intrauterine contraceptive devices as compared to non-users. Lancet 1976;2:221-4.
34. Osser S, Liedholm P, Sjoberg NO. Risk of pelvic inflammatory disease among users of intrauterine devices, irrespective of previous pregnancy. Am J Obstet Gynecol 1980;138:864-7.
35. Dahling JR, Weiss NS, Metch BJ, et al. Primary tubal infertility in relation to the use of an intrauterine device. N Engl J Med 1985;312:937-41.
36. Sweet RL, Draper D, Hadley WK. Etiology of acute salpingitis: influence of episode number and duration of symptoms. Obstet Gynecol 1981;58:62-8.
37. Svensson L, Westrom L, Ripa KT, et al. Differences in some clinical and laboratory parameters in acute salpingitis related to culture and serologic findings. Am J Obstet Gynecol 1980;138:1017-21.
38. Platt R, Rice PA, McCormack WM. Risk of acquiring gonorrhea and prevalence of abnormal adnexal findings among women recently exposed to gonorrhea. JAMA 1983;250:3205-9.
39. Paavonen J. *Chlamydia trachomatis* in acute salpingitis. Am J Obstet Gynecol 1980;138:957-9.
40. Ripa KT, Svensson L, Treharne JD, et al. *Chlamydia trachomatis* infection in patients with laparoscopically verified acute salpingitis. Results of isolation and antibody determinations. Am J Obstet Gynecol 1980;138:960-4.
41. Eschenbach DA, Buchanan TM, Pollock HM, et al. Polymicrobial etiology of acute pelvic inflammatory disease. N Engl J Med 1975;293:166-71.
42. Sweet RL, Draper DL, Schachter J, et al. Microbiology and pathogenesis of acute salpingitis as determined by laparoscopy: what is the appropriate site to sample? Am J Obstet Gynecol 1980;138:985-9.
43. Henry-Suchet J, Catalan F, Loffredo V, et al. Microbiology of specimens obtained by laparoscopy from controls and from patients with pelvic inflammatory disease or infertility with tubal obstruction: *Chlamydia trachomatis* and *Ureaplasma urealyticum*. Am J Obstet Gynecol 1980;138:1022-5.
44. Watts DH, Eschenbach DA. Treatment of chlamydia, mycoplasma, and group B streptococcal infections. Clin Obstet Gynecol 1988;31:435-52.
45. Berman SM, Harrison HR, Boyce WT, et al. Low birth weight, prematurity, and postpartum endometritis. Association with prenatal cervical *Mycoplasma hominis* and *Chlamydia trachomatis* infections. JAMA 1987;257:1189-94.
46. Brunham RC, Binns B, McDowell J, et al. *Chlamydia trachomatis* infection in women with ectopic pregnancy. Obstet Gynecol 1986;67:722-6.
47. Hager WD, Eschenbach DA, Spence MR, et al. Criteria for diagnosis and grading of salpingitis. Obstet Gynecol 1983; 61:113-4.
48. Jacobson L, Westrom L. Objectivized diagnosis of acute pelvic inflammatory disease. Am

J Obstet Gynecol 1969;105:1088.
49. Sweet RL, Mills J, Hadley KW, et al. Use of laparoscopy to determine the microbiologic etiology of acute salpingitis. Am J Obstet Gynecol 1979;134:68-74.
50. Curran JW. Economic consequences of pelvic inflammatory disease in the United States. Am J Obstet Gynecol 1980; 138:848-51.
51. Sweet RL. Diagnosis and treatment of salpingo-oophoritis. Mediguide to Obstet Gynecol 1983:2:1-6.
52. Centers for Disease Control. Sexually transmitted disease treatment guidelines. MMWR 1985;34:Suppl 45: USPHS.
53. Stamm WE, Guinan ME, Johnson C, et al. Effect of treatment regimens for *Neisseria gonorrhoeae* on simultaneous infection with *Chlamydia trachomatis*. N Engl J Med 1984;310:545-9.
54. Washington AE, Browner WS, Korenbrot CC. Cost-effectiveness of combined treatment for endocervical gonorrhea. Considering co-infection with *Chlamydia trachomatis*. JAMA 1987;257:2056-60.
55. Sweet RL, Schachter J, Robbie MO. Failure of beta-lactam antibiotics to eradicate *Chlamydia trachomatis* in the endometrium despite apparent clinical cure of acute salpingitis. JAMA 1983;250:2641-5.
56. Centers for Disease Control. Antibiotic-resistant strains of *Neisseria gonorrhoeae:* policy guidelines for detection, management, and control. MMWR 1985;36:Suppl 5:USPHS.
57. Spence MR. The treatment of gonorrhea, syphilis, chancroid, lymphogranuloma venereum, and granuloma inguinale. Clin Obstet Gynecol 1988;31:453-65.
58. Bush LM, Boscia JA. Disseminated multiple antibiotic-resistant gonococcal infection: needed changes in antimicrobial therapy. Ann Intern Med 1987;107:692-3.
59. Sweet RL, Gibbs RS. Sexually transmitted diseases. In: Infectious diseases of the female genital tract. Baltimore: Williams and Wilkins, 1985:17-52.
60. Martens MG, Berkeley AS, Faro S, et al. Efficacy of ofloxacin versus cefoxitin plus doxycycline in the outpatient treatment of pelvic inflammatory disease. Eur Cong Clin Microb, 1989. abstract 43/PP3.
61. Hager WD, Pascuzzi M, Vernon M. Efficacy of oral antibiotics following parenteral antibiotics for serious infections in obstetrics and gynecology. Obstet Gynecol 1989;73:326-9. abstract.

CHAPTER 5

Recent Advances in Outpatient Therapy of Urinary Tract Infections

Joseph R. Dalovisio, M.D.
New Orleans, Louisiana

INTRODUCTION

Because urinary tract infections (UTIs) occur frequently and may lead to chronic renal insufficiency in certain patients, these infections are an important medical problem. Although treatment of UTI may be considered a mundane, straightforward topic, recent investigations into criteria for diagnosis of UTI, identification of new urinary pathogens, studies of briefer lengths of treatment, and development of newer antimicrobial agents have led us to reconsider strategies for treatment of UTI. Certain patients previously treated with seven to ten days of oral antibiotics can now be treated with single-dose oral therapy.[1] Selected patients previously hospitalized for treatment of pyelonephritis may now be treated as outpatients with intravenous (IV) or oral therapy due to development of antimicrobial agents with extended spectrums and serum half-lives, as well as to availability of new outpatient health care delivery systems. These trends toward shorter treatment and outpatient therapy are compatible with the current emphasis on less costly health care.

LOWER URINARY TRACT INFECTION

Lower urinary tract infections (acute cystitis) are usually characterized in adult females by symptoms of dysuria, frequency, fever and flank pain; systemic symptoms tend to be absent. Urine cultures have been the mainstay for diagnosing UTIs. In the past, voided urine specimens showing greater than 10^5 colonies/ml of *Enterobacteriaceae* in adults were considered as definitive diagnosis of a UTI. However, the bacteriologic criteria for diagnosing UTIs has been complicated by the realization that pathogens newly recognized in the urinary tract — such as coagulase-negative staphylococci and *Chlamydia trachomatis*, and older pathogens, including group D streptococci and some *Enterobacteriaceae* — may have colony counts 10^2 to 10^5 colonies/ml and still be responsible for a UTI. Platt has shown that women with dysuria and pyuria indicating UTI may have "significant" urine bacterial colony counts of 10^2 colonies/ml.[2]

Women with acute onset of frequency and dysuria with less than 10^5 organisms/ml of urine have been termed as having "acute urethral syndrome."[3] Causes for this include bacterial cystitis with low counts, vaginitis, genital herpes, and urethral infection with *C. trachomatis*, *Ureaplasma urealyticum*, or *Neisseria gonorrhoeae*. Evaluation of sexually active patients with acute urethral syndrome should include pelvic examination and tests or treatment for *Chlamydia* and *N. gonorrhoeae*.

Urine microscopy is mandatory in the evaluation of patients with suspected lower UTI. Pyuria is the most important finding suggestive of UTI as it is absent in only 1% of asymptomatic, non-bacteriuric patients.[4] Bacteriuria can also be estimated by urine microscopy. An initial urine culture need not be done as its cost-effectiveness is doubtful for otherwise healthy female patients presenting typical cystitis symptoms and compatible urine microscopy showing pyuria and bacteriuria.[5] Urine cultures should be performed in patients with anatomically abnormal urinary tracts, or with underlying systemic diseases placing them at increased risk for pyelonephritis, or with multiple prior courses of antibiotics causing concern about antibiotic resistance.

A number of tests to distinguish upper tract urinary infection from lower tract infection have been used in the past. These usually include ureteral catheterization with culture, bladder wash-out test, and renal biopsy. None of these are practical or indicated in the routine management of a UTI. More recently, the antibody-coated bacteria test has been used, but problems with the sensitivity and specificity of this test have diminished its usefulness.[6] Clinical parameters such as the presence of fever, nausea, vomiting, and flank or abdominal pain remain the most useful signs suggesting upper from lower tract infection. A significant number of women with only lower tract symptoms may have upper tract infection also. Successful treatment with single-dose oral therapy is a useful predictor of lower tract infection *(vide infra)*.

Since 1976 a number of publications have reported results of trials in which a single dose of an antibiotic was given for a UTI. Because many antibiotics are excreted at high concentrations in the urine and because bladder infection is a superficial mucosal infection, it follows that a brief burst of a high concentration of antibiotics might be curative. However, the situation with cystitis is entirely different than that with pyelonephritis or prostatitis where invasive parenchymal infection has occurred, and penetration or activity of the antibiotics might be suboptimal. A review of the subject of single-dose treatment of a UTI points out that 12 of 14 studies reported single-dose treatment to be as effective as traditional regimens.[7] Deficiencies of currently available studies and objectives of future studies on single-dose UTI therapy have been discussed by Fihn and Stamm.[8]

Single-dose therapy appears to have potential advantages of lower cost, improved patient compliance, and decreased side effects. It should not be used in patients with structural abnormalities of the urinary tract including indwelling catheters, patients with a high probability of renal infection, and patients with impairment of renal function. In women without the above risk factors, a trial of single-dose therapy is indicated. Preferred regimens are trimethoprim 320 mg plus sulfamethoxazole 1600 mg (two double-strength tablets) or amoxicillin 3 gm. If symptoms persist beyond four days, then repeat urinalysis and culture are indicated. If persistent infection is documented, then the patients should be treated with 14 days of therapy with an antimicrobial to which the pathogen is susceptible. Useful agents for UTI include sulfisoxazole, amoxicillin, trimethoprim, trimethoprim/sulfamethoxazole, cephalexin, doxycycline, nitrofurantoin, and the newer quinolones, norfloxacin and ciprofloxacin. A follow-up culture to establish cure should be performed one to two weeks after discontinuation of antibiotics. Rubin has pointed out that a high percentage of patients failing single-dose treatment may also fail "conventional" therapy (10-14 days), and many of these patients will have functional or structural abnormalities of the urinary tract.[9] Patients failing 14-day treatment regimens should have a urologic evaluation and should then be treated for six weeks with an antibiotic to which the organism is susceptible.

Male patients, because of the possibility of prostatitis, and female patients with the possibility of subclinical pyelonephritis should be treated *initially* with seven days of an antibiotic to which the organism is susceptible and re-evaluated with culture after discontinuation of antibiotic treatment. These recommendations are based partly on available studies and partly on my opinion. Definitive answers regarding many aspects of UTI management are not available and there remains a wide diversity of opinion regarding duration of treatment and appropriate follow-up for UTI.

UPPER URINARY TRACT INFECTION

Patients with a clinical diagnosis of pyelonephritis are frequently admitted to hospitals for the initial part of the treatment course. This permits close monitoring of the patient response to treatment, which is initially often intravenous. Also, IV therapy circumvents problems of absorption of orally administered medication from the GI tract. Patients known to be unlikely to take medicines as prescribed and patients with underlying diseases such as renal stone disease, diabetes mellitus and neoplastic disease should be admitted to the hospital for treatment. For patients with concomitant illnesses hospital admission allows for prompt intervention, both diagnostically and therapeutically, if clinical response is not as good as expected.

OUTPATIENT TREATMENT OF PYELONEPHRITIS

In the last few years financial pressures have forced health care systems to reduce cost. Alternate schemes of treatment have been developed. Selected patients with pyelonephritis might be treated out of the hospital. Appropriate treatment could include administration of IV or IM antibiotics at home by home health nurses on a daily or several times daily basis, daily visits by patients to the physician's office for once-daily IM or IV antibiotics, or oral therapy with some of the newer, potent, broad-spectrum oral antibiotics like the fluoro-4-quinolones. In addition to financial advantages of outpatient therapy, many patients prefer to be treated on an outpatient basis for personal, family or social reasons.

CEPHALOSPORINS

The development of several new cephalosporins with serum half-lives compatible with once-daily dosing intervals and with broad enteric gram-negative rod spectrums has been helpful for outpatient parenteral treatment of UTI.

Cefonicid

Cefonicid is a second-generation cephalosporin very similar in bacteriologic spectrum to cefamandole. It has a half-life of 4.5 hours, compatible with a dosing interval of every 24 hours. It is excreted 98% unchanged in the urine. Average urine concentrations after a one-gram dose are 1308 mcg/ml at 0 to 2 hours and 149 mcg/ml at 12 to 24 hours.[10] Organisms are considered susceptible if their minimal inhibitory concentration (MIC) is < 8 mcg/ml. Its spectrum of urinary pathogens includes most strains of *Escherichia coli, Klebsiella, Proteus mirabilis, Enterobacter aerogenes, Citrobacter, Providencia rettgeri,* coagulase-negative staphylococci and *N. gonorrhoeae*. It is not active against most strains of *Pseudomonas aeruginosa, Providencia vulgaris, Providencia morganii,* and enterococci. The usual dosage for pyelonephritis is one gram IM or IV every 24 hours. Cefonicid could be used for once-daily IV or IM therapy of pyelonephritis if *P. aeruginosa*, enterococci, *P. vulgaris*, or *P. morganii* are not a serious risk. Adverse effects are infrequent and mainly include local irritation from injection, elevated liver function, or hypersensitivity. The current cost of one gram of cefonicid to the pharmacy at our institution is about $13.

Ceftriaxone

Ceftriaxone is a third-generation cephalosporin with a serum half-life of six to eight hours, consistent with a once-daily dosing schedule. Serum trough levels at 24 hours are approximately 9 mcg/ml after 1 gm IV or 15 mcg/ml after 2 gm IV.[11] Urine concentrations of ceftriaxone after 1 gm IV are 132 mcg/ml at 12 to 24 hours and 32 mcg/ml at 24 to 48 hours. After a 2 gm dosage, urine concentrations of ceftriaxone are 198 mcg/ml at 12 to 24 hours and 40 mcg/ml at 24 to 48 hours. Organisms are considered susceptible if the MIC is less than or equal to 16 mcg/ml. Ceftriaxone (3.6 ml per gm) is well absorbed after intramuscular injection, which may be painful unless diluted with lidocaine. From one-third to two-thirds of injected ceftriaxone is excreted in the urine unchanged, and the balance is excreted by the biliary tract. The microbiologic spectrum of this agent includes most of the *Enterobacteriaceae, N. gonorrhoeae,* and coagulase-negative staphylococci. The activity of ceftriaxone against *P. aeruginosa* is variable. Currently, at the Ochsner Medical Institutions, only 25% of strains of *P. aeurginosa* are susceptible. As with other cephalosporins, ceftriaxone is inactive against enterococci. The safety profile of this agent is similar to other cephalosporins. Adverse effects include hypersensitivity reactions, diarrhea, and suprainfections, especially with yeasts and enterococci. The dosage is 1 or 2 gm IM or IV once daily. The cost of this drug is about $23 per gram to the pharmacy at our institution. Thus, although it is a broader-spectrum drug than cefonicid, it is also more costly per day. It could be used cost-effectively for once-daily IV or IM treatment of pyelonephritis where risk of a resistant *P. aeruginosa* or enterococcus was not present.

OTHER PARENTERAL ANTIBIOTICS

A variety of other antibiotics could be given parenterally two or more times daily on an outpatient basis, but the delivery of these types of drugs with every 12-hour to every 4-hour dosage schedules becomes logistically prohibitive and increasingly costly with increasing frequency of administration. In addition, the use of a drug like amikacin, gentamicin, or tobramycin carries risk of oto- or nephrotoxicity, as well as increased cost for monitoring renal function and serum antibiotic levels, thus diminishing their utility in the outpatient setting.

ORAL THERAPY FOR PYELONEPHRITIS

In the past, oral therapy for pyelonephritis was usually restricted to patients with mild illness. The development of broader-spectrum oral agents with activity against most *Enterobacteriaceae* and *P. aeruginosa* has made oral treatment for pyelonephritis more feasible. The risk of a resistant gram-negative rod with a tissue concentrating quinolone such as ciprofloxacin is very low. A Gram's stain of the urine should be done in all patients with pyelonephritis in order to define the morphology of the infecting organism. Gram-positive diplococci are likely to be group D streptococci (enterococci) and should be treated with oral amoxicillin or IV ampicillin in the non-penicillin allergic patient. In patients with penicillin allergy, therapy should be initiated with IV vancomycin.

In a penicillin-allergic patient with mild pyelonephritis and gram-positive diplococci on Gram's stain of the urine, norfloxacin or ciprofloxacin can be used for therapy with close clinical follow-up. Patients with pyelonephritis where Gram's stain of the urine shows gram-negative rods can be treated initially with ciprofloxacin, with a high probability that the organism will be susceptible. Other oral agents that concentrate in genitourinary tract tissue and that have broad gram-negative spectrums but less breadth than ciprofloxacin include trimethoprim/sulfamethoxazole, amoxicillin/clavulanate, and cefuroxime axetil. The decision whether to treat a patient with oral versus parenteral therapy depends on the clinician's assessment of a variety of previously mentioned factors including likelihood of compliance, potential absorptive problems (including vomiting), poor prognostic factors related to underlying illness and general degree of illness. If clinical experience with the quinolones in treatment of pyelonephritis continues to be favorable, it is likely that sicker patients currently treated parenterally will be treated increasingly with oral therapy.

QUINOLONE ANTIBIOTICS

The development of the fluoro-4-quinolone family of antibiotics is probably the most significant advance in outpatient antibiotic therapy in recent years. A void in the antibacterial spectrum of our oral antimicrobial armamentarium has existed for years in the areas of the more resistant *Enterobacteriaceae* and *P. aeruginosa*, all of which are important uropathogens. The high urinary levels, good safety profile, and good absorption after oral administration make flouro-4-quinolones particularly attractive for therapy of UTI.

The quinolones are analogs of nalidixic acid with a quinolone ring in place of a 1,8 napthyridine ring. A l-piperazinyl group at the 7 position gives anti-pseudomonal activity, and this activity is augmented by a fluorine atom at the 6 position. The mechanism of action, although not completely understood, is related to the molecule's inhibition of DNA gyrase, an enzyme that repairs bacterial DNA and maintains it in a supercoiled state in the cell. Development of resistance to the fluoro-4-quinolones seems to occur less frequently than to nalidixic acid.[12] Cross-resistance among the quinolones may occur, but cross-resistance with other classes of antibiotics is uncommon.[13]

In general, the fluoro-4-quinolones have broad activity against *E. coli, Klebsiella pneumoniae, Enterobacter, Serratia marcescens, Salmonella, Shigella, Campylobacter,*

P. mirabilis, Moraxella, P. aeruginosa, N. gonorrhoeae, and staphylococci.[14] Anaerobes, *Pseudomonas cepacia,* and *Pseudomonas maltophila* are usually resistant.[14] The streptococci are generally intermediate in susceptibility.[14] Many enterococci are inhibited by urinary levels of the fluoro-4-quinolones.[14] While a large number of fluoro-4-quinolones are being developed, only two products are currently commercially available in the United States; thus, remarks will be limited to these two compounds: norfloxacin and ciprofloxacin.

Norfloxacin

Norfloxacin was the first of the fluoro-4-quinolones released commercially in the United States. It is only 30% to 40% absorbed after oral administration. Peak serum level after a 400 mg dose in normal subjects is approximately 1.5 mcg/ml.[15]

FIGURE 1. Serum (●) and blister-fluid (o) levels of norfloxacin after oral administration of a 400 mg dose. Vertical bars indicate standard deviation (from reference 15)

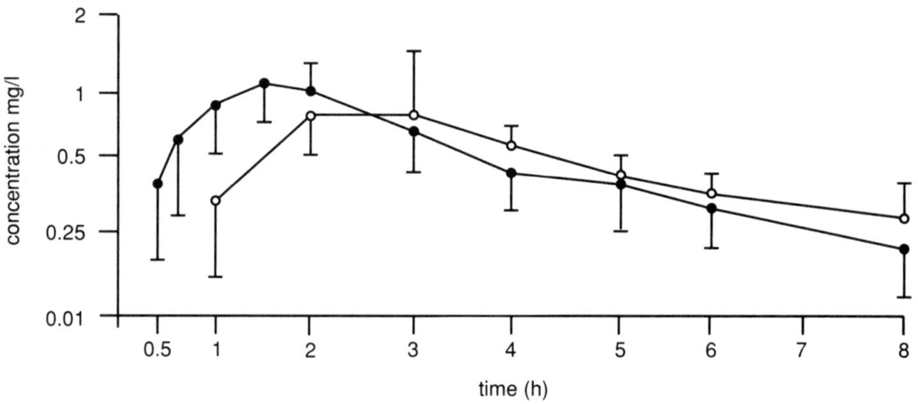

Twenty-five to forty percent of the parent drug is excreted in the urine, resulting in urine norfloxacin levels of 200 mcg/ml or more. Prostate tissue levels after two 400 mg doses are 2.5 mcg/gm of tissue. In adults with normal renal function, the usual dosage of norfloxacin is 400 mg every 12 hours. In patients with creatinine clearances of less than 20 ml per minute, dosage is usually 400 mg once daily. Hemodialysis does not affect elimination. In a large study of *in vitro* susceptibilities, the MIC_{50} (concentration of antibiotics required to inhibit 50% of stains) for *S. aureus, E. coli, E. cloacae, S. marcescens,* and *P. aeruginosa* were all less than 1 mcg/ml. The MIC_{50} for *Streptococcus faecalis* was 3.13 mcg/ml. The MIC_{90} (concentration of antibiotics required to inhibit 90% of stains) for *E. coli* was 0.2 mcg/ml, for *E. cloacae* 0.78 mcg/ml, for *S. aureus* and *P. aeruginosa* 3.13 mcg/ml, for *S. faecalis* 6.25 mcg/ml and for *S. marcescens* 12.5 mcg/ml.[14] Urinary pathogens are considered susceptible to norfloxacin if the MIC is <16 mcg/ml and resistant if the MIC is >32 mcg/ml.

The most common adverse effects occurring with norfloxacin are nausea (2.8%), headaches (2.7%), and dizziness (1.8%). Central nervous system effects such as seizures and myoclonus have been reported with norfloxacin and other quinolones, but cause and effect have not been established. The most frequent laboratory abnormalities observed with norfloxacin are eosinophilia (1.8%), elevated SGOT and SGPT (1.8%), elevated alkaline phosphatase (1.4%), and decreased WBC (1.2%).[16]

Ciprofloxacin

Ciprofloxacin is 83% absorbed after an oral dose. Peak serum level of ciprofloxacin in normal volunteers is 2 to 3 mcg/ml after a 500 mg dose.[15,17]

FIGURE 2. Serum (●) and blister-fluid (o) levels of ciprofloxacin after oral administration of a 500 mg dose. Vertical bars indicate standard deviation (from reference 15)

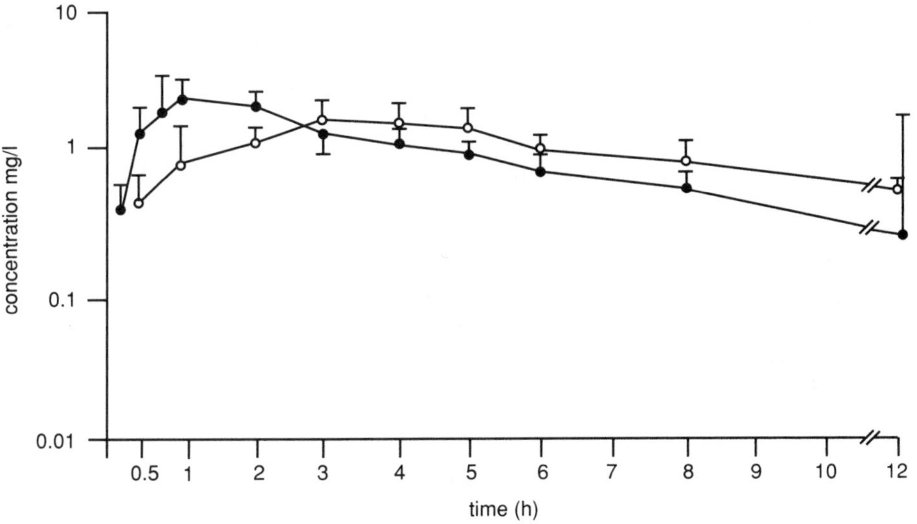

Twenty-five to forty percent of the parent drug is excreted unchanged by the kidneys. Urine ciprofloxacin levels usually exceed 200 mcg/ml. Ciprofloxacin levels in prostatic secretions were 3 mcg/ml 12 hours after a single 500 mg dose in one study.[18] Dosage for ciprofloxacin in patients with UTI with normal renal function is 250 mg to 500 mg every 12 hours. Renal failure has less effect on serum ciprofloxacin levels than on norfloxacin levels, but some modification of dosage is recommended in patients with creatinine clearances of less than 50 ml per minute, with a dose of from 250 mg to 500 mg every 12 to 24 hours. Hemodialysis has only a modest effect on elimination of ciprofloxacin.

With ciprofloxacin the MIC_{50} for *E. coli* and *E. cloacae* is <0.05 mcg/ml, for *S. marcescens* and *P. aeruginosa* 0.2 mcg/ml, for *S. aureus* 0.39 mcg/ml, and for *S. faecalis* 0.78 mcg/ml. The MIC_{90} for *E. coli* is 0.1 mcg/ml, for *E. cloacae* 0.2 mcg/ml, for *P. aeruginosa* and *S. aureus* 0.78 mcg/ml, for *S. faecalis* 1.56 mcg/ml and for *S. marcescens* 6.25 mcg/ml.[14] Thus, compared to norfloxacin, ciprofloxacin tends to have lower MICs for comparable organisms and higher serum levels at currently recommended doses. Susceptibility breakpoints for ciprofloxacin proposed by the National Committee for Clinical Laboratory Standards can be considered "susceptible" if the MIC is <1 mcg/ml and "resistant" if the MIC is >2 mcg/ml.[17] These levels appear to be correlated more to systemic than to urinary infection, since much higher ciprofloxacin levels than these would be achieved in the urine.

Several important drug interactions occur with ciprofloxacin. Administration of theophylline with ciprofloxacin can elevate serum theophylline levels.[17] Also, probenecid raises serum ciprofloxacin levels by blocking renal tubular excretion.[17]

Ciprofloxacin, as with other quinolones, is generally well tolerated. The most frequent adverse effects reported were nausea (5.2%), diarrhea (2.3%), vomiting (2%), abdominal pain (1.7%), headache (1.2%), restlessness (1.1%), and rash (1.1%).[17] Ciprofloxacin may be associated with central nervous system side effects like tremor, hallucinations, or seizures and therefore should be used with caution in patients predisposed to convulsive disorders.

Laboratory abnormalities most commonly associated with ciprofloxacin include elevated SGPT (1.9%), elevated SGOT (1.7%), elevated alkaline phosphatase (0.8%), elevated LDH (0.4%), eosinophilia (0.6%), leukopenia (0.4%), and elevated creatinine (1.1%).[17] Crystalluria has also been reported.

A fairly large number of patients have been treated with norfloxacin and ciprofloxacin in comparative studies with both uncomplicated and complicated UTI (underlying anatomical or functional abnormalities of the urinary tract or acute pyelonephritis). These are well summarized by Malinverni and Glauser.[19] In uncomplicated UTI, norfloxacin or ciprofloxacin was at least as effective as trimethoprim/sulfamethoxazole or amoxicillin and more effective than nalidixic acid or nitrofurantoin. Data on single-dose treatment with the quinolones are too limited to draw conclusions. Several randomized comparative trials of norfloxacin or ciprofloxacin with other agents in complicated UTI have shown these agents to be at least as effective as amoxicillin or trimethoprim/sulfamethoxazole.[19] Only a small number of patients have been studied comparing quinolones with a parenteral aminoglycoside with or without a concomitant beta-lactam drug in complicated UTI. One study showed that norfloxacin cured more patients than did parenteral treatment, but the results may have been hampered by an inadequate follow-up period for all patients.[20] A few reports of noncomparative trials of ciprofloxacin or norfloxacin in UTI caused by *P. aeruginosa* look promising, but variability in underlying conditions, dosages, duration of treatment, and length of follow-up complicate conclusive analysis of the data.[19] In clinical studies of treatment of UTI, emergence of resistance has been observed infrequently among organisms other than *P. aeruginosa.* The magnitude of resistance with *P. aeruginosa* is unknown at the present time. The effectiveness of the quinolones in treatment of UTI in patients with varying degrees of renal failure is also unknown.

Importantly, problems with quinolone toxicity in experimental animals include arthropathy in juvenile joints and nephropathy from crystalluria at high doses. Because of the concern over adverse effects on developing cartilage, none of the quinolones are approved for usage in children or pregnant women.[16]

Antacids containing magnesium hydroxide and aluminum hydroxide may interfere with absorption of all quinolones and therefore should not be given concomitantly. Since food may decrease absorption, norfloxacin should be given one hour before meals or two hours after meals.

BACTERIAL PROSTATITIS

Acute Bacterial Prostatitis

Acute bacterial prostatitis is usually characterized by fever, low back or perineal pain, and symptoms of bladder irritability. The infection is usually caused by coliform organisms or enterococci. Patients treated with antimicrobials that concentrate in the urine and to which the uropathogen is susceptible are usually cured, even if the antimicrobials fail to penetrate well into prostatic secretions.

Chronic Bacterial Prostatitis

Chronic bacterial prostatitis may be asymptomatic or may present with symptoms of low back or perineal pain. Fever is unusual. Chronic bacterial prostatitis may be diagnosed as relapsing UTI (because of the uropathogen's persistance in the prostate). Because of the difficulty in eradicating chronic bacterial prostatitis, antibiotic penetration into the prostate may be a more important factor than with acute prostatitis. Tetracycline, including doxycycline, trimethoprim and erythromycin have all been shown to penetrate fairly well into prostatic secretions.[21] Because of the excellent penetration and bacteriologic spectrum of norfloxacin and ciprofloxacin into the prostate, they would seem ideal candidates for treatment of prostatitis. A summary of the data in the relatively small number of studies that have looked at success rates of quinolone therapy for prostatitis shows success rates of 63% to 92%.[19]

CONCLUSION

In summary, single-dose treatment for lower tract UTI is advantageous in areas of cost, compliance, and adverse effects and may be of some diagnostic value in separating upper from lower urinary tract infections. Development of the fluoroquinolones and once-daily parenteral cephalosporins, ceftriaxone and cefonicid, has now allowed selected patients with complicated UTI to be treated as outpatients. Many questions related to optimal duration of treatment of UTI, appropriate follow-up, and the roles and limitations of the fluoroquinolones remain yet to be answered.

REFERENCES

1. Fihn SD, Johnson C, Roberts P, et al. Trimethoprim - sulfamethoxazole for acute dysuria in women: a single dose or 10-day course. Ann Intern Med 1988;108:350-7.
2. Platt R. Quantitative definition of bacteriuria. Am J Med 1983;75(1B):44-52.
3. Stamm WE, Wagner KF, Amsel R, et al. Causes of the acute urethral syndrome in women. N Engl J Med 1980;303:409-15.
4. Stamm WE. Measurement of pyuria and its relation to bacteriuria. Am J Med 1983;75(1B):53.
5. Ronald AR, Conway B. An approach to UTI in ambulatory women. In: Remington JS, Swartz MN, eds. Current clinical topics in infectious diseases. New York: McGraw-Hill, 1987:9:77-125.
6. Nicolle L, Ronald A. Recurrent UTI in adult women: diagnosis and treatment in infectious disease. Infect Dis Clin North Am Dec 1987.
7. Philbrick JT, Bracikowski JP. Single dose antibiotic treatment for uncomplicated UTI. Less for less? Arch Intern Med 1985;145:1672.

8. Fihn SD, Stamm WE. Interpretation and comparison of treatment studies for uncomplicated UTI in women. Rev Infect Dis 1985;7:468.
9. Rubin RH. Single dose therapy of UTIs. In: Neu H, ed. Infectious diseases. New York: Eugene Schuessler, 1984:14:4-12.
10. Smith Kline & French Laboratories. Monocid[R] product monograph. Philadelphia, 1984.
11. Roche scientific summary: the clinical evaluation of Rocephin.[R] Nutley, New Jersey: Hoffman LaRoche Laboratories, 1986:138.
12. Neu H. Bacterial resistance to fluoroquinolones. Reviews of Infect Disease 1988;10(Suppl 1):557-63.
13. Rubinstein E, Segv S, Lev B. The 4-quinolones: A promising new class of antibiotics. Hospital Therapy Aug 1986;39-66.
14. Mitsuhashi S. Comparative antibacterial activity of new quinolone-carboxylic acid derivatives. Rev Infect Dis 1988:10(Suppl 1):527-31.
15. Wise R, Griggs D, Andrew JM. Pharmacokinetics of the quinolones in volunteers: a proposed dosing schedule. Rev Infect Dis 1988: 10(Suppl 1):S83-9.
16. Noroxin Package insert. Lansdale: Merck Sharp & Dohne, Jan 1988.
17. Miles, Inc. Compendium of preclinical and clinical data. In: Ciprofloxacin product information monograph. New York: Marcel Dekker, Inc., 1988.
18. Dalhoff A, Weidner W. Diffusion of ciprofloxacin into prostatic fluid. Eur J Clin Microbiol 1984;3:360-2.
19. Malinverni R, Glauser MP. Comparative studies of fluoroquinolones in the treatment of UTI. Rev Infect Dis 1988;10(Suppl 1):S153-63.
20. Cherubin C, Stilwell S. Norfloxacin vs. parenteral therapy in the treatment of complicated UTI. Scand J Infect Dis 1986;48(Suppl1):32-7.
21. Colleen S, Mardh P. Prostatitis. In: Holmes KK, Mardh P, Sparling PF, et al, eds. Sexually transmitted diseases. New York: McGraw-Hill, 1984:662-71.

CHAPTER 6

Outpatient Antimicrobial Therapy of Skin and Skin Structure Infections

George A. Pankey, MD
New Orleans, Louisiana

There are 193 living species of monkeys and apes. One hundred and ninety-two of them are covered with hair. The exception is the naked ape, self-named *Homo sapiens*.

—Desmond Morris

INTRODUCTION

This chapter is concerned with the outpatient management of primary and secondary bacterial infections of the skin and skin structure. Important viral infections of the skin are covered in the chapter on sexually transmitted diseases. A discussion of fungal infections of the skin and nails falls outside the scope of this chapter and book.

THE SKIN AS A NATURAL BARRIER

The skin is a complex organ comprised of the following layers: epidermis (stratum-corneum and malpighii layer), basement membrane zone, and dermis. In fact, the epidermis is an excellent barrier, being rarely penetrated by microorganisms. Only the openings of the pilosebaceous apparatus, which include the hair follicles, interrupt its continuity. In addition, the normal physical and chemical composition of the skin contributes to its ability to minimize the number of microorganisms on its surface. Its relative dryness represses the growth of most pathogenic bacteria and fungi, particularly gram-negative bacilli, and the acidic pH and complex lipids in sebaceous secretions of the skin are believed to play an inhibitory role by affecting the metabolism of many microorganisms. In addition, the process of desquamation, in which an epidermal cell layer is replaced approximately every month, continually removes attached bacteria.

The Colonization Process

Bacterial colonization of the skin begins shortly after birth, with microorganisms that are commonly referred to as "resident" and "transient" flora. Resident microorganisms have the ability to survive and multiply under normal skin conditions, but are most likely to be found in the body folds, such as the gluteal cleft, axillae, nail folds, toe webs, and openings of the hair follicles. As would be expected, primary skin infections occur most frequently in these areas. Bacteria primarily found in the resident flora include *Staphylococcus epidermidis*, aerobic and anaerobic *Corynebacteria*, and anaerobic staphylococci and streptococci. Gram-negative bacilli including *Escherichia coli*, and species of *Proteus*, *Enterobacter*, *Pseudomonas*, and *Acinetobacter* may be part of the resident flora in the most moist areas of the skin. The role of the resident flora in inhibiting other microorganisms is unclear, but they may serve as additional defense mechanisms against invasion of the skin by more serious microorganisms.

Transient microorganisms, on the other hand, are those deposited on the skin via the environment, including those from the infectious discharges of the skin and respiratory tract of another person, from contaminated objects or from an individual's own mucous membranes. *Staphylococcus aureus*, *E. coli*, *Bacillus* species, *Neisseria* species, and some streptococci may colonize the skin for brief periods. Some individuals carry potentially pathogenic bacteria, such as *S. aureus*, in the nasal and/or anal mucosa and contaminate other skin areas from that site.

Whether or not species of the resident or transient flora produce disease depends on the number and virulence of the bacteria present, as well as on the local and systemic defenses of the host. Any violation of the intact epidermis, be it from cold, heat, chemicals, bites, stings or other trauma (accidental or surgical), may be associated with an infection.

Types of Infections

Skin lesions associated with infectious diseases generally fall into six categories. Primary infections, including impetigo, folliculitis, furuncles, carbuncles, and cellulitis associated with trauma, and secondary infections are most common. Other lesions occur as a result of hematogenous spread (ecthyma gangrenosum associated with *Pseudomonas aeruginosa* bacteremia, etc.), direct extension (sinus tract from an osteomyelitic bone, etc.), dermatotoxin (toxic shock syndrome, scarlet fever, etc.), or hypersensitivity reaction (erythema nodosum, etc.).[1]

DIAGNOSIS

Most primary and secondary bacterial infections involving the cutaneous structures have a typical appearance, with the patient giving a typical history. Therefore, therapy can be prescribed without the need for an expensive laboratory evaluation involving a culture and *in vitro* antimicrobial susceptibility studies. If purulent material is available, a Gram's stain examination should allow one to diagnose streptococci (gram-positive diplococci or cocci in chains), staphylococci (large gram-positive cocci, singular or in clusters) or gram-positive and gram-negative bacilli.

TREATMENT FOR PRIMARY INFECTIONS

Impetigo

Cultures are not indicated in patients with impetigo unless they are performed for the purpose of epidemiologic evaluation or because of failure of response. A systemic antimicrobial may be necessary only for patients who fail to respond to a topical antimicrobial, such as mupirocin 2% ointment. Mupirocin is active against both penicillinase-producing and methicillin-resistant *S. aureus*. In addition to its use in therapy for impetigo, mupirocin can be applied to the nasal mucosa four times daily for one week in patients who are nasal carriers of *S. aureus*.[2] Mupirocin is not active against *Enterobacteriaceae*, *P. aeruginosa* or fungi, and emergence of resistant staphylococci has been reported with long-term topical therapy. Only a trace amount is absorbed into the systemic circulation, and this is rapidly hydrolyzed.[3] Crusted impetigo with streptococci on the Gram's stain will respond to ten days of therapy with penicillin V or erythromycin, even when penicillin-resistant *S. aureus* is cultured from the specimen. Bullous impetigo is usually due to *S. aureus*, against which a number of antimicrobials are effective, even for penicillinase-producing strains. Appropriate antibiotics for treatment of bullous impetigo include amoxicillin/clavulanate, cefadroxil, cephalexin, ciprofloxacin, cloxacillin, dicloxacillin, erythromycin and trimethoprim/sulfamethoxazole. The agent chosen is determined by patient drug allergy and tolerance, as well as by cost considerations. If strains of methicillin-resistant *S. aureus* are prevalent in a community, ciprofloxacin 500 mg-700 mg q 12h or trimethoprim/sulfamethoxazole 160/800 q 12h should be used.

Folliculitis

Folliculitis is most often caused by staphylococci or *P. aeruginosa* (whirlpool or spa associated).[4] Folliculitis usually responds to cleansing of the entire body at least once daily using antibacterial soap, with special attention to all hairy areas. Severe cases may be treated with an oral antimicrobial given for up to five days. Cloxacillin or erythromycin for staphylococcal folliculitis, and ciprofloxacin for *P. aeruginosa* folliculitis, are reasonable choices. If external otitis and subnipple breast infection occurs with *P. aeruginosa* folliculitis, systemic therapy with ciprofloxacin 500-750 mg every 12 hours for ten days should be given.

S. auereus folliculitis may be relatively asymptomatic but can progress to a furuncle or, rarely, a carbuncle. Incision and drainage of furuncles and carbuncles may be curative; but in order to decrease the chance of having staphylococci released into the bloodstream, possibly causing infection at a distant site such as in the endocardium or bone, I prefer to administer simultaneously an antimicrobial such as cefadroxil 500-1000 mg every 12 hours for seven to ten days, with the first dose given 30-60 min prior to any incision and drainage procedure. In an immunocompetent patient, no culture is necessary unless erythromycin is used, or less the patient is from a geographic area where a high percentage of the *S. aureus* are methicillin-resistant.

Recurrent Furunculosis

Recurrent furunculosis requires incision and drainage of fluctuant lesions, prolonged antimicrobial therapy, application of mupirocin 2% ointment to the nasal mucosa, maintenance of good hygiene, and avoidance of predisposing conditions, such as tight clothing, excessive sweating, and contamination of the skin with oil (such as might be experienced by a service station attendant). Some patients with recurrent furunculosis require several weeks of therapy with an antimicrobial, such as cefadroxil 500-1000 mg every 12 hours or cloxacillin 250 mg every six hours. For the beta-lactam allergic patient, ciprofloxacin 500-750 mg every 12 hours or erythromycin 500 mg every six hours is appropriate. Rifampin 300 mg q 12h may be added to the first ten days of therapy in patients in whom infections recur.

Cellulitis

Needle tissue aspirations have been attempted in the bacteriologic diagnosis of patients with lower extremity cellulitis, but the yield of bacteria is unfortunately too low to recommend the procedure.[5,6] Occasionally, a punch biopsy of the leading edge of the cellulitis will yield the organism on culture. However, this procedure is unnecessary, since most cellulitis will respond to therapy directed at the presumed bacterial pathogens on the basis of the clinical aspects. For example, nail puncture-wound cellulitis of the foot is most likely due to *P. aeruginosa*. These patients should all have surgical debridement and ciprofloxacin 750 mg q 12h until the microbiological diagnosis is established. Patients with servere cellulitis of the lower leg should receive an antimicrobial that is active against both *S. aureus* and Group A beta-hemolytic streptococci, such as cefazolin IM or IV. In mild-to-moderate cases, cefadroxil taken orally is usally adequate. Erythromycin and vancomycin (in mild and moderate cases, respectively) are alternatives for cephalosporin-allergic patients.

In patients with lower leg cellulitis associated with *Tinea pedis*, culture of the toe web at the site of the most advanced area usually results in many different bacteria being isolated. If Group A beta-hemolytic streptococci are isolated, this organism is likely the pathogen for the cellulitis.

Other Common Primary Skin Infections

Other common primary skin infections include paronychia, ecthyma and lymphangitis. *S. aureus* and/or Group A beta-hemolytic streptococci are the usual pathogens. If no systemic illness is apparent, these infections almost always respond to appropriate surgical and oral antimicrobial therapy.

TREATMENT FOR SECONDARY INFECTIONS

Skin disorders, such as atopic eczema, psoraisis and neurodermatitis, may become colonized or secondarily infected with *S. aureus* and/or other bacteria. A positive culture would not necessarily confirm the microbiological diagnosis of a secondarily infected area. Therefore, secondary infection is a clinical diagnosis that fortunately is typically associated with a favorable response to antimicrobial therapy. However, unless the primary skin problem resolves, recolonization with bacteria usually occurs and, at some point, may again produce secondary infection. Antimicrobials used for bullous impetigo are also usually effective for these types of secondary infections.

Cutaneous Infections Following Trauma

Secondary cutaneous infections associated with traumatic injury also can be difficult to diagnose bacteriologically. Involved bacteria may be part of the resident and transient flora, as well as being present in the soil, water, etc. associated with the original injury. Also, infections following trauma are affected by a number of factors involving both local and systemic defenses. Infection is most likely to result if there is devitalized or necrotic tissue, inadequate local circulation (atherosclerosis, thrombosis, etc.), foreign materials in the wound (dirt, wood, chemicals), hematoma or seroma, obesity, a delay in treatment of more than four hours, or the presence of multiple wounds. Systemic factors favoring the development of infection include dehydration, malnutrition, advanced age, obesity, infection at a site remote from the traumatized tissue, diabetes mellitus (uncontrolled), uremia, cirrhosis, malignancy, and any type of immunosuppressive therapy, such as glucocorticoid therapy.

Treatment of these infections includes extensive debridement of all devitalized tissue, drainage of any purulent material that develops, and administration of antimicrobial(s). The antimicrobial(s) initially chosen should be active against the resident skin flora, as well as against bacteria associated with the material contaminating the injured skin.

CUTANEOUS INFECTIONS FOLLOWING SURGERY

Surgical Wound Infections

In general, surgical wound infections that occur within 24 to 48 hours are due to Group A beta-hemolytic streptococci or *Clostridium perfringens* and should be treated in the hospital. On the other hand, *S. aureus, S. epidermidis* and aerobic and strict anaerobic gram-negative bacilli wound infections occur four or more days after surgery, with surgical (incision, drainage, debridement) and antimicrobial therapy frequently occurring in the outpatient setting.

Initial antimicrobial therapy is decided on the basis of a Gram's stain, with possible modification after *in vitro* susceptibility of the isolate(s) is known. Occasionally, rapidly-growing mycobacterial wound infections *(Mycobacterium fortuitum and Mycobacterium chaelonei)* do not manifest until weeks after surgery. These infections require surgical debridement and long-term (weeks to months) therapy with the following antimicrobials in various combinations, depending on susceptibility testing: amikacin, cefoxitin, ciprofloxacin, doxycycline, and trimethoprim/sulfamethoxazole.

Specific Problems Following Aortocoronary Bypass Procedures

The extensive practice of aortocoronary bypass procedures using saphenous vein grafts has resulted in occasional leg cellulitis at the vein donor site. The infection may not be manifested until the patient has been discharged from the hospital, despite the fact that most frequently the bacteria involved are beta-hemolytic streptococci (A, B, C, or G groups). Prolonged oral antimicrobial therapy is indicated as recurrence is not unusual.

S. aureus can produce cellulitis at the vein donor site, although isolated abscesses along the surgical incision are more likely areas for this organism. A reasonable choice for these types of infection is cefadroxil or erythromycin for beta-lactam-allergic patients. In the case of cellulitis I prefer three weeks of therapy rather than the ten days usually judged as adequate for staphylococcal abscess.

Sternal wound infections after aortocoronary bypass usually do not manifest clinically until after the patient is discharged from the hospital, and they are most likely due to *S. aureus, S. epidermidis, P. aeruginosa, Serratia* or rapidly growing *Mycobacteria*. Ciprofloxacin is the only oral agent active against most strains of all of these bacteria; it is administered 750 mg every 12 hours in conjunction with appropriate incision, drainage, and debridement.

Catheter Site Infection

The tissues around Hickman and other catheters for vascular or peritoneal access can become infected with bacteria similar to those found in sternal wound infections. In many areas, *S. aureus* and *S. epidermidis* are resistant to all penicillins and cephalosporins, so that therapy with oral fluoroquinolones (ciprofloxacin, ofloxacin, etc.), trimethoprim/sulfamethoxazole or intravenous vancomycin is necessary. In many cases, removal of the catheter is <u>not</u> required; however, if the catheter is maintained, at least three weeks of antimicrobial therapy is necessary.

CHRONIC SKIN INFECTIONS

Outpatient management of chronic skin structure infection represents a major challenge. Most of these cases are infected pressure sores (decubitus ulcers) or involve the lower extremities and are a result of secondary infection following a break in the skin of a patient with diabetes mellitus, arterial insufficiency, venous stasis, vasculitis or hematologic problems, such as sickle-cell anemia, leukemia or dysproteinemia.

As expected, the increase in decubitus problems has parallelled the growth of the elderly population. In fact, there is now a journal, *Decubitus*, concerned with nothing but pressure sores. In addition to treatment of the infectious component with surgical abridement and antimicrobials, good nutrition and relief of pressure are of paramount importance for healing in these patients, as well as in those with lower extremity infection. If patients with infections of pressure sores or of the lower extremities are to be managed initially at home, there must be: (1) recent onset of infection; (2) minimal or no drainage; (3) no gangrene; (4) no fever or toxicity; and (5) a reliable patient or attendant(s).

Diagnostic Considerations

In all types of chronic lower extremity and pressure sore infections, a Gram's stain and culture of purulent material or an aspirate for both aerobic and anaerobic bacteria are important. Culture of open, ulcerated lesions may not yield the true pathogen, but antimicrobial therapy directed at the isolated bacteria is usually effective.[9] Rarely, primary infection with fungi or mycobacteria is associated with chronic leg ulcers, and biopsy of tissue for special stains and cultures is required. Radiologic examination for tissue gas and osteomyelitis is useful. In diabetic patients with foot and leg ulcer infections, it is important to maintain debridement with whirlpool treatments. Also, since most of these patients have *Tinea pedis*, a topical antifungal agent should be used routinely between the toes and on any involved areas of the feet. Some patients require oral ketoconazole therapy for control of their fungal infection.

Antimicrobial Treatment of Pressure Sores

Pressure sores (decubitis ulcers) are almost invariably secondarily infected with two or more bacterial species. Aerobes and strict anaerobes are usually present, and as the final results of cultures may not be available for five or more days, initial antimicrobial therapy of such infections must be empiric. Common pressure sore pathogens that are aerobic include *Proteus mirabilis*, *Staphylococci* (*aureus* and *epidermidis*), *E. coli*, *Klebsiella*, *Pseudomonas*, and Groups A, B, and D streptococci. Important strict anaerobic bacteria include *Bacteroides* species, *Clostridium* species, *Peptococcus* species, *Peptostreptococcus*, *Eubacterium* and *Propionibacterium*.[7,8] Two good empiric oral antimicrobial regimes are ciprofloxacin 750 mg q 12h plus metronidazole 1 gram q 12h or clindamycin 600 mg q 8h.

Lower Extremity Infections

The management of lower extremity infections is similar to that of decubitus ulcers. It is important to determine the underlying cause and modify the contributing factors, if possible. This involves attempting to improve the vascular supply to the involved area with relief of pressure, as well as using angioplasty or bypass surgery for arterial insufficiency, and is absolutely imperative if any antimicrobial therapy is to be effective. Control of local and surrounding cellulitis with debridement and antimicrobial(s) is important, but maintenance of good nutrition is essential for healing. Some patients with pressure sores or leg ulcers require skin grafting when the infection is controlled. Frequently, resolution requires weeks or months of therapy. Many patients cannot be treated initially at home but can soon be discharged from the hospital and moved home or to a nursing facility.

A crepitant skin structure infection usually means a strict anaerobic bacterium is involved, but *E. coli* and some other facultatively anaerobic bacteria may produce gas in tissues, especially in diabetic patients with lower extremity infections. Patients with crepitant cellulitis frequently have peripheral blood leukocytosis and blood cultures positive for one or more of the bacterial species seen on the Gram's stain of the drainage. A foul-smelling lesion indicates a strict anaerobe(s) is involved. These conditions are surgical emergencies, with antimicrobials playing an important secondary role. All patients with these conditions should be hospitalized for parenteral therapy with broad-spectrum antimicrobials.[10]

SKIN INFECTIONS SECONDARY TO BITES

Bacteria associated with cellulitis following dog, cat or human bites are shown in Table I. Tetanus immunity should be assured in all patients whether bitten or not. Rabies immune globulin and vaccine may be indicated following animal bites.

Most infections following cat bites are due to *Pasteurella multocida*, a gram-negative bacillus that is also associated with infections following dog bites. *S. aureus* not only is carried by animals but also occurs on the skin of bitten patients and may be carried into the wound resulting in an infection. Antimicrobial therapy for seven to ten days with amoxicillin/clavulanate potassium 500 mg q 8h or doxycycline 100 mg q 12h is usually effective for cellulitis following animal (including human) bites. *P. multocida* is resistant to cloxicillin, cephalexin, cefaclor, cefadroxil, and erythromycin; *Eikenella corrodens*, an occasional pathogen associated with infections secondary to human bites, is resistant to clindamycin. Therefore, these agents, as well as those with no activity against anaerobic bacteria, should not be used for initial therapy of infections following animal bites. If amoxicillin/clavulanate potassium or doxycycline in full doses can be administered within two to four hours of the bite, most cellulitis can be prevented with only two days of treatment. In penicillin-allergic and tetracycline-intolerant patients, good alternatives are ciprofloxacin 500-750 mg q 12h plus metronidazole 1 gm q 12h or clindamycin 600 mg q 8h.

TABLE I. Bacterial infection following bites (from reference 5)

Type of Bite	Dog	Cat	Human
Pasteurella multocida	+	+	0
Dysgonic fermenter (DF-2)	+	+	0
S. aureus	+	+	+
Streptococci	+	+	+
Anaerobes	+	+	+
Eikenella corrodens	0	0	+

SKIN INFECTIONS ASSOCIATED WITH WATER CONTAMINATION

Breaks in the skin following trauma contaminated with water do not usually become infected with microorganisms present in the water. If infection occurs, it is more likely to be due to *S. aureus* present on the skin at the time of trauma. Water-borne bacteria that may produce infection in skin structure include gram-negative bacilli (*Vibrio, Aeromonas, Pseudomonas,* etc.), gram-positive bacilli (*Erysipelothrix*) and acid-fast bacilli (*Mycobacterium marinum*).

Vibrio vulnificus and *Aeromonas hydrophilia* result in infections that frequently require extensive surgical debridement. *Vibrio vulnificus* infections are most likely to occur in patients immunocompromised by liver disease who are injured in salt water. I believe that if appropriate antimicrobial therapy could be started within a few hours of trauma, many of these infections could be prevented. Ciprofloxacin and doxycycline appear to be oral agents with the most *in vitro* activity, and ciprofloxacin is active against *Aeromonas* as well.

Mycobacterium marinum causes skin infections following abrasions or puncture wounds occurring in all types of aquatic environments, including swimming pools and aquariums. These lesions are most commonly seen on the hand. After several weeks of incubation, the infection may manifest as a flat, red macular area that disappears without specific therapy, or may progress to form a nodule or lesion with ulceration. Infection may spread in the lymphatics, producing visible red nodules mimicking lymphocutaneous sporotrichosis. Diagnosis is confirmed by biopsy of the margin of the skin lesion, which usually shows a granulomatous response. Direct acid-fast smear of the biopsy tissue and culture for mycobacteria at 30-32° C is recommended.

Antimicrobial treatment is indicated for all patients in whom the diagnosis of *Mycobacterium marinum* infection is made, since it is unpredictable which lesions will clear without therapy. Treatment is usually given for a minimum of three months following initial surgical debridement of any subcutaneous tissue involvement. Rifampin plus ethambutol or, alternatively, doxycycline, minocycline or trimethoprim/sulfamethoxazole have all been used successfully.

SKIN INFECTIONS ASSOCIATED WITH SOIL CONTAMINATION

In addition to *S. aureus*, a potential pathogen in all traumatic wounds, infections associated with contaminated soil are particularly prone to involve unusual microorganisms, such as *Bacillus cereus*, *Nocardia* and rapidly growing mycobacteria. In addition to thorough cleaning and debridement of soil contaminated wounds, it is advisable to give antimicrobials in an attempt to prevent the development of infection. This is most likely to be successful if administered within two to four hours of the trauma. Trimethoprim/sulfamethoxazole 160/800 mg plus metronidazole 1 gm both given every 12 hours for 48 hours is a good choice. Ciprofloxacin 750 mg q 12h also for 48 hours is used for treatment of puncture wounds of the feet to prevent *P. aeruginosa*, cellulitis and osteomyelitis. If longer than four hours has elapsed since the injury, I would recommend seven days of preventive treatment.

ROUTES OF ADMINISTRATION

Outpatient antimicrobial therapy for skin and skin structure infections may be administered intramuscularly, intravenously or orally. In addition, in Europe and Japan, antimicrobial rectal suppositories have been studied and are available for such drugs as metronidazole. Rectal suppositories would represent a means of administering therapy to patients who are nauseated and wish to receive treatment where parenteral therapy is not available. Rectal suppositories of ceftriaxone are presently being evaluated, and plasma concentrations following 500 mg rectal suppository are 10 micrograms per ml eight hours later which, although lower than following 500 mg of IV infusion, still represents an over ninety times the MIC for 90% of tested strains of Group A and Group B streptococci, *Streptococcus pneumoniae, Hemophilus, Neisseria gonorrhoeae* and *Neisseria meningitidis*. The trough level at eight hours is equal to or exceeds the MIC for 90% of tested *S. aureus, E. coli, Klebsiella, Morganella,* and *Serratia*.[11] Obviously, the use of antimicrobial rectal suppositories in pediatrics as well as in adult patients, who cannot take oral medications, would eliminate the inconvenience and cost of parenteral therapy.

CONTINUING PROBLEMS

Some continuing problems with outpatient antimicrobial therapy of bacterial skin structure infections include: (1) the fact that there is no effective single oral antimicrobial for microorganisms associated with some polymicrobic (aerobic and anaerobic) infections; (2) elimination of the nasal and/or anal carriage of *S. aureus* in patients with recurrent staphylococcal skin-structure infections; (3) intolerance of antimicrobials by the patient (gastrointestinal rashes, etc.); (4) unavailability of antimicrobial rectal suppositories; and (5) expense of administration of intravenous agents.

REFERENCES

1. Pankey GA, Katner HP, Valainis GT, et al. Overview of bacterial infections of the skin and soft tissue and clinical experience with ticarcillin plus clavulanate potassium in their treatment. Am J Med 1985;79:Suppl 5B:106-15.
2. Casewell MW, Hill RLR, Duckworth GJ. Elimination of nasal carriage of methicillin resistant *Staphylococcus aureus* with muciprocin during a hospital outbreak. J Antimicrob Chemother 1988;22:377-84.
3. Mupirocin—A new topical antibiotic. The Medical Letter; 1988;30:55-6.

4. Price D, Ahearn DG. Incidence and persistence of *Pseudomonas aeruginosa* in whirlpools. J Clin Microbiol 1988; 26(9):1650-4.
5. Hook EW III, Hooton TM, Horton CA, et al. Microbiologic evaluation of cutaneous cellulitis in adults. Arch Intern Med 1986;146:295-7.
6. Newell PM, Norden CW. Value of needle aspiration in bacteriologic diagnosis in cellulitis in adults. J Clin Microbiol 1988;26(3):401-4.
7. Longe RL. Current concepts in clinical therapeutics: pressure sores. Clin Pharm 1986;5:669-81.
8. Mulder GD, LaPan M. Decubitus ulcers: update on new approaches to treatment. Geriatrics 1988;43:37-49.
9. Wheat LJ, Allen SD, Henry M, et al. Diabetic foot infections. Arch Intern Med 1986;146:1935-40.
10. Pankey GA. Approach to rashes and infections of the skin and subcutaneous tissues including infected bites and marine infections. In: Kelley WM, ed. Textbook of internal medicine. Philadelphia: J.B. Lippincott Co., 1989:2:1725-9.
11. Personal Communication, Roy Clelland, Roche Laboratories.

CHAPTER 7

Outpatient Management of Osteomyelitis in a DRG Era

Layne O. Gentry, M.D.
Houston, Texas

INTRODUCTION

Epidemiology

Adult osteomyelitis is now diagnosed more often in patients who have experienced severe bone trauma or who have had elective placement of an orthopedic prosthesis or appliance. In adults, a diagnosis of acute osteomyelitis, defined as the signs and symptoms of bone infection present for less than one month, is most often limited to complications of IV catheters or IV substance abuse. Chronic osteomyelitis, defined as the presence of signs and symptoms of osteomyelitis for more than one month, is usually accompanied by drainage from one or more sinus tracts.

Although the difference in diagnosis between acute and chronic osteomyelitis relates to the duration of symptoms, there is a great distinction made between these two forms of osteomyelitis in terms of patient management and prognosis. The acute form of osteomyelitis occurs most often in children and is seen frequently as a complication of the hematogenous dissemination of *Staphylococcus aureus* to bone during a bacteremia. The acute form responds readily to antibiotic therapy. On the other hand, chronic osteomyelitis is usually a complication of exposure of open wounds and fractures to gram-positive skin flora and gram-negative flora, bacteria that are encountered by a patient in critical care areas during a hospitalization.

While the incidence of acute osteomyelitis has been confined, the incidence of chronic osteomyelitis has been increasing. Within the past ten years, the number of cases due to nosocomial gram-negative organisms and mixed gram-positive/gram-negative infections has risen.[1-4] Unfortunately, many of these nosocomial infections are due to pathogens resistant to traditional antimicrobial agents.

An analysis of the osteomyelitis literature between 1967 and 1985 reveals that there is a trend towards fewer cases where *S. aureus* or *Streptococcus* sp. are the single isolate and a trend towards more gram-negative, enterococcal, polymicrobial and mixed infections (Table I.). Most of the cases reported were in patients hospitalized for acute trauma, who subsequently developed post-traumatic osteomyelitis, often at the site of the trauma. Many other patients developed osteomyelitis following an orthopedic procedure. This epidemiologic data suggests that nosocomial pathogens such as *Pseudomonas aeruginosa*, *Serratia marcescens* and *Enterobacter* sp. will increasingly be involved in osteomyelitis.

TABLE I. Post-traumatic osteomyelitis - 1967-1985 - etiology

Pathogen/percent	1967 (1)	1970 (2)	1971 (3)	1985 (4)
Staphylococcus aureus %	68	29	58	32
Gram-negative rods	12	29	27	25
Mixed Gram- neg/pos	20	20	4	33
Streptococcus sp.	-	13	11	7
Others (incl. anaerobes)	-	9	-	3

Trend Towards Ambulatory Care

Because of recent constraints applied by third-party payers, in particular the diagnosis-related group (DRG) system of reimbursement implemented by Medicare, there is a need for an early and specific diagnosis for osteomyelitis, in order that outpatient or home care management might be effective. Under the 1988 DRG classification as seen in Table II, a patient with confirmed osteomyelitis is allowed 10.7 days of hospitalization to achieve a cure. If bone biopsy and surgical debridement are required, 8.4 days are allowed; and 3.5 days are allowed for simple surgical debridement.

TABLE II. Medicare DRG for osteomyelitis, 1988 (from US Government)

DRG No.	Explanation	No. of Days	Amt Paid
238	Medical diagnosis of osteo	10.7	$5,196.00
231	Osteo w/ surgical debridement	3.5	$2,615.00
216	Osteo w/ bone biopsy and surgical debridement	8.4	$5,006.51

However, there have been no significant breakthroughs in the standard treatment regimen of 42 days of parenteral antibiotics for osteomyelitis. Hospitals obviously cannot afford to treat osteomyelitis patients on an inpatient basis for a prolonged period of time; therefore, there is a strong incentive to discharge osteomyelitis patients as soon as possible and to complete the antibiotic administration on an outpatient or home-care basis.

Unlike many serious or life-threatening infections, chronic osteomyelitis is not usually associated with impaired mental function or physical debilitation, apart from the infected bone. A great majority of osteomyelitis patients are capable of resuming normal activity and an employment schedule while under antibiotic care for their infection.

The focus, then, of the following, is to outline for the practicing physician a reasonable approach to the early diagnosis and outpatient management of osteomyelitis in the adult patient.

DIAGNOSIS

Sinus Tract Culture

Because most cases of chronic osteomyelitis are associated with sinus tract drainage, and because this discharge may be easily cultured by a swab sample, it would be ideal if this material would yield an accurate diagnosis of the bacterial etiology of the associated osteomyelitis. Unfortunately, research indicates that this is not the case. In a recent study of 72 patients with osteomyelitis, summarized in Table III, the overall specificity of sinus tract cultures was 86%, and its sensitivity was 76%, compared to a specificity of 100% and a sensitivity of 85% for bone biopsy.[5]

TABLE III. Comparison of bone biopsy with sinus tract culture (from reference 5)

	Specificity	Sensitivity
Bone Biopsy (n=72)		
All patients		0.86
All organisms		0.85
S. aureus	1.00 (by defn)	0.93
other GPC	1.00	0.76
P. aeruginosa	1.00	0.91
other GNR	1.00	0.77
	Specificity	**Sensitivity**
Sinus Tract		
All patients	0.83	0.75
All organisms	0.86	0.76
S. aureus	0.90	0.70
other GPC	0.69	0.65
P. aeruginosa	0.75	0.82
other GNR	0.96	0.88

Reliance upon sinus tract cultures as a guide for empiric therapy offers the risk that overly broad spectrum antibiotic therapy may be initiated, with corresponding increased risks for emergence of resistance and adverse reactions if combination therapy is chosen. Biopsy of the infected bone, either open or percutaneous, is the only accurate method of determining the precise bacterial etiology of osteomyelitis.

The use of the special biopsy needle designed by Craig[6] has led to the introduction of bone biopsy under fluoroscopic control, performed on an outpatient basis with a minimum of pain. Multiple cultures should be performed with histopathologic examination, in order to minimize the likelihood of a false-negative result.

Radiographic Techniques

Conventional radiographic techniques, including computed tomography (CT), are widely used in the diagnosis of osteomyelitis.[7-12] The main drawback to radiographic techniques in diagnosis is a lack of sensitivity early in the infectious process. Most radiographic techniques are not diagnostic until three to four weeks after infection.

Magnetic resonance imaging (MRI) is the newest radiographic technique, and by far the most sensitive. MRI measures tissue water, and can detect minute differences in the water content in adjacent tissues. Because inflammation and tissue edema are common in the early stages of infection, MRI can detect the difference between inflamed tissue and bone, as compared to normal bone, which has little to no detectable water. Usually, MRI is used diagnostically involving the vertebral body and osteomyelitis of the spine.[13] However, MRI is the most expensive and least readily available of the radiographic techniques, and further studies are needed to confirm its relevance for osteomyelitis apart from the spine.

Radionuclide Scans

Radionuclide scans using technetium-99 polyphosphate (Tc-99) complexes were the first to detect evidence of bone infection. Tc-99 binds to crystal surfaces and areas of osteoblastic bone activity. The ability to detect early changes in blood flow in bone offers the possibility of early diagnosis of osteomyelitis. However, both false-positive and false-negative results have been reported with Tc-99 scans, especially in post-trauma and post-operative patients.[14] Therefore, it is necessary to confirm Tc-99 scans with the histopathology and microbiology from an open or needle biopsy.

Gallium-67 citrate (Ga-67) scans have been used to identify areas of osteomyelitis in bone, and this scan has been shown to be more sensitive than Tc-99 scans.[15] Unfortunately, the specificity of Ga-67 scans is relatively poor, and, given the size of the field and the resolution of the instrumentation, the sensitivity in small bones can suffer because of the insignificant number of acute inflammatory cells that uptake the Ga-67.

Recently, the Indium-111 leukocyte (In-III) scan has been shown to be more specific than the other scans, because indium-labelled white cells from the patient are allowed to migrate under chemotaxis into the area of bone inflammation and infection; there is also evidence that the In-111 scan may be the most sensitive of the radionuclide techniques.[16] However, it must be noted that all radionuclide scans have difficulty distinguishing infection from either infarction or tumor necrosis.

TREATMENT

Surgical Debridement

The presence of sequestered bone and accumulated inflammatory debris in areas of chronic osteomyelitis is extremely common. Because of the tissue's devascularized nature, bacteria may thrive, and bacterial contamination has been the most significant prognostic factor in determining the success or failure of antibiotic therapy for our patients. In fact, many published studies have indicated that inadequate surgical debridement with the resultant availability of devascularized tissue has caused the majority of treatment failures. It is, therefore, essential that a combined medical-surgical approach be initiated for the management of the patient with osteomyelitis.

Antibiotic Selection and Therapy

A six-week regimen of parenteral antibiotic(s), with antibiotic(s) selected as a result of culture and sensitivity data obtained via bone biopsy, remains the standard therapy for chronic osteomyelitis. Difficulties associated with long-term intravenous access have been alleviated through the widespread use of the subcutaneous, skin-tunnelled catheter of Broviac.[17] This catheter allows easy access for up to two years without the significant risks of catheter sepsis associated with percutaneous insertion. Of note, all patients in our center who require long-term intravenous access have surgical implantation of this catheter.

For cases of osteomyelitis due to *S. aureus*, the beta-lactamase resistant penicillins such as nafcillin or oxacillin remain the therapy of choice. Although in children with *S. aureus* osteomyelitis, a shorter course of parenteral antibiotics followed by a longer regimen of oral antibiotics has been successful; parenteral therapy alone appears to be effective in adults.[18] In the United States and Europe, there has been an increase in the isolation of methicillin-resistant strains of *S. aureus*.[19] Although these pathogens are often sensitive to cephalosporins *in vitro*, these patients usually fail on cephalosporin therapy.[20] Vancomycin remains the only reliable and effective treatment for osteomyelitis due to methicillin-resistant *S. aureus*.

Antibiotic selection is often complicated by the increasing incidence of mixed infections. Nosocomial gram-negative bacteria are frequently resistant to many of the common broad-spectrum antibiotics; in particular, resistant strains of *P. aeruginosa*, *S. marcescens* and *E. cloacae* are not uncommon in cases of osteomyelitis. For this reason, the specific culture and sensitivity data obtained via the bone biopsy is essential to the selection of appropriate antibiotics.

The use of the newer beta-lactams as monotherapy has been investigated recently. Some of the results of clinical trials at our center and affiliated institutions are presented in Table IV. The rate of clinical success ranged from 68% for imipenem/cilastatin to 100% in the few patients who received aztreonam. Clinical failures were most often due to inadequate surgical debridement with recurrence of infection associated with persistent sequestrum. Although less frequent, emergence of resistance for the causative pathogen was noted in each study. Overall, the beta-lactams are associated with a high degree of clinical success and minimal adverse experiences related to drug therapy, despite the prolonged regimen.

TABLE IV. Newer antimicrobial agents as therapy (from Gentry LO, published and unpublished data)

Drug	n	Cure(%)	Improve *	Fail
Cefotaxime	84	73 (87)	-	11 (13)
Ceftazidime	122	100 (82)	10 (8)	12 (10)
Ceftizoxime	33	25 (76)	-	8 (24)
Ceftriaxone	104	72 (69)	10 (10)	22 (21)
Aztreonam	11	11 (100)	-	-
Imipenem/Cilastatin	34	23 (68)	-	11 (32)

We have recently compared the efficacy and safety of oral ciprofloxacin with standard parenteral therapy for osteomyelitis, and these data are presented in Table V.[21] While parenteral therapy, either a penicillin and aminoglycoside combination or a third generation cephalosporin, usually required six weeks, regimens of eight weeks or longer were not uncommon with oral ciprofloxacin. Overall, the two approaches were remarkably similar in clinical and bacteriologic efficacy. Because of the economic and patient care advantages of orally administered antibiotics, the FDA has recently approved oral ciprofloxacin as monotherapy for osteomyelitis due to susceptible organisms. However, at our center we have found a need for increased microbiologic diligence during oral ciprofloxacin therapy, because of concerns over emergence of resistance.

TABLE V. Oral ciprofloxacin versus parenteral therapy (from reference 21)

	Oral Cipro	IV
Clinical Responses		
Number of Evaluable Patients	31	28
Successes	24 (77%)	22 (79%)
Failures	7 (19%)	6 (21%)
at End of Therapy	1 (3%)	1 (3%)
at Follow-up (12 mo)	6 (19%)	5 (18%)
Those With Adverse Reactions	1 (3%)	4 (14%)
Superinfections	4 (13%)	2 (7%)
Bacteriologic Responses		
Number of Pathogens Isolated	40	40
S. aureus	9 (22%)	11 (27%)
other gram-positive	2 (2%)	5 (12%)
P. aeruginosa	12 (29%)	5 (12%)
other gram-negative	17 (46%)	19 (49%)
Eradication-End of RX	39 (98%)	39 (98%)
Persistence-End of RX	1 (2%)	1 (2%)

Economic Considerations

There are tremendous economic incentives for home-care treatment of osteomyelitis with oral antibiotics. The analysis in Table VI shows that, excluding all laboratory and microbiology charges, which are identical for all treatment modalities, total inpatient care for osteomyelitis using a third-generation cephalosporin via Broviac catheter may cost $13,700. Substituting home care for inpatient care results in a savings of $7,820. The further substitution of an oral quinolone for the third-generation cephalosporin results in an additional savings of $4,930. The more economical home care with an oral quinolone costs only 8% of the cost of inpatient care with a third-generation cephalosporin, roughly $1,000, exclusive of laboratory charges.

TABLE VI. Economic considerations and antibiotic selection

Inpatient versus Outpatient (six weeks of therapy)	
42 days hospital room @ $200 per day	$ 8,400.00
42 clinic visits @ $60 per visit	2,520.00
Savings Attributable to Outpatient Care	$ 5,880.00
Outpatient versus Home Care	
42 clinic visits @ $60 per visit	$ 2,520.00
8 home visits @ $50 per visit, 3 clinic visits	580.00
Further Savings Attributable to Home Care	$ 1,940.00
Parenteral versus Oral Therapy	
Six-week supply, third generation cephalosporin*	$ 3,500.00
Six-week supply, oral quinolone	370.00
Credit for no Broviac catheter insertion	1,800.00
Savings Attributable to Oral Quinolones	$ 4,930.00

** includes IV administration supplies*
prices those of St. Luke's Episcopal Hospital, Houston, TX, 1988

Patient Management

Patients with osteomyelitis are usually stable, and require only infrequent attention from the attending physician. Those receiving home care for intravenous administration of antibiotics should be visited by a nurse once each week, for an inspection of the catheter site, a review of the technique, and an inventory of supplies including medication, heparin for anticoagulation and disposables.

Laboratory tests are performed at two-to four-week intervals, depending on age, renal function and the toxicity of the antibiotics used. Tests include white blood cell count and differential, serum creatinine and erythrocyte sedimentation rate. The WBC and differential allow for early detection of allergic reactions, indicated by eosinophilia, and for the correction of anemia as indicated by a low hemoglobin. Serum creatinine monitors kidney function, which must be watched closely if an aminoglycoside is included in the therapeutic regimen. Because the ESR test is very nonspecific, the downward trend toward normal is the only positive prognostic finding. Routine radiographs and radionuclide scans are not necessary, except at four-to six-month intervals for follow-up.

Parenteral therapy is usually stopped after six weeks, yet the duration of therapy with oral quinolones may be significantly longer. Clinical observations that indicate a good prognosis include closure of the sinus tract, decrease in erythema and swelling, and radiographic evidence of healing. However, these improvements will occur only gradually.

An early return to a full range of motion is the key to rehabilitation in cases of osteomyelitis. Unless there is the danger of a pathologic fracture due to the destruction of bone resulting from the infection and surgical debridement, patients should maintain a normal schedule of activities.

CONCLUSION

We conclude that there are strong economic and patient care incentives to outpatient management of osteomyelitis. Although there are procedures that somewhat enhance our diagnostic capabilities, such as radiography and radionuclide scans, open or percutaneous bone biopsy is essential to an accurate diagnosis of osteomyelitis and appropriate selection of antibiotics. Intravenous therapy remains the standard, yet the early successes of the oral fluoroquinolones, as well as the recent introduction of newer oral cephalosporins, offer the prospect of further advances in economical patient care.

REFERENCES

1. Clawson DK, Dunn AW. Management of common bacterial infections of bones and joints. J Bone Joint Surg 1967; 49:164-82.
2. Gerszten E, Allison MJ, Dalton HP. An epidemiologic study of 100 consecutive cases of osteomyelitis. Southern Med J 1970; 63:365-7.
3. Waldvogel FA, Medoff G, Swartz MN. Treatment of osteomyelitis. N Engl J Med 1970;283:822.
4. Gentry LO. The role of newer beta-lactam antibiotics in the treatment of osteomyelitis. Am J Med 1985;78:134-9.

5. Self PL, Gentry LO. Correlation of bone biopsy and sinus tract culture in osteomyelitis. In: Programs and abstracts of the 25th ICAAC. 1985: Abstr No. 896.
6. Craig FS. Vertebral body biopsy. J Bone Joint Surg 1956; 78:218-24.
7. Kuhn JP, Berger PE. Computed tomographic diagnosis of osteomyelitis. Radiology 1979;130:503-6.
8. Hermann G, Rose JS. Computed tomography in bone soft tissue pathology of the extremities. J Comput Assist Tomogr 1979; 3:58-66.
9. Ram PC, Martinez S, Korobkin M, et al. CT detection of intraosseous gas: a new sign of osteomyelitis. AJR 1981;137:721-3.
10. Larde D, Mathieu D, Frija J, et al. Vertebral osteomyelitis disk hypodensity on CT. AJR 1982;139:963-7.
11. Kattapuram SV, Phillips WC, Boyd R. CT in pyogenic osteomyelitis of the spine. AJR 1983;140:1199-201.
12. Wing VW, Brooke JR, Federle MP, et al. Chronic osteomyelitis examined by CT. Radiology 1985;154:171-4.
13. Smith FW. Nuclear magnetic resonance (NMR) imaging in the diagnosis of spinal osteomyelitis. Magnetic Resonance Imaging 1984;2:53-6.
14. Lisbona R. Observations on the sequential use of Tc-99 phosphate complex and Ga-67 imaging in osteomyelitis, cellulitis and septic arthritis. Esiol 1977;123:123.
15. Kolyvas E, Rosenthal L, Ahronheim GA, et al. 67 Ga-citrate imaging during treatment of acute osteomyelitis in childhood. Clin Nucl Med 1978;3:461-6.
16. Rapropoulos V, Doherty PW, Goss TP, et al. Acute osteomyelitis: advantage of white cell scans in early detection. AJR 1982;139:1077-82.
17. Broviac JW, Cole JJ, Scribner BH. A silicone rubber atrial catheter for prolonged parenteral alimentation. Surg Gynecol Obstet 1973;136:602-6.
18. Nelson JD. A critical review of the role of oral antibiotics in the management of hematogenous osteomyelitis. In: Remington JS, Swartz MN, eds. Curent clinical topics in infectious disease. New York: McGraw-Hill, 1983:4:64-74.
19. Crossley KB, Ross J. Colonization of hospitalized patients by *Staphylococcus aureus, Staphylococcus epidermidis* and *Enterococci*. J Hosp Infect 1985;6:179.
20. Fekety R. The management of the carrier of methicillin-resistant *Staphylococcus aureus*. In: Remington JS, Swartz MN, eds. Current clinical topics in infectious disease. New York: McGraw-Hill, 1987:8:169-80.
21. Gentry LO, Gomez GR. Oral ciprofloxacin compared with parenteral antibiotics in the treatment of osteomyelitis. Antimicrob Agents Chemother (in press).

CHAPTER 8

Special Problems of Infants and Children

Jerome O. Klein, M.D.
Boston, Massachusetts

INTRODUCTION

Physicians responsible for the care of infants and children should consider a number of recent advances in outpatient use of antimicrobial drugs for treatment and prevention of infections particularly common in children. Three areas in which many of these advances have occurred are: management of the febrile child with occult bacteremia; treatment and prevention of otitis media; and treatment of other upper respiratory illness.

NEW DRUGS

Outpatient Management of the Febrile Child with Risk Features of Occult Bacteremia

Management of the febrile child with risk features of occult bacteremia has been the subject of considerable interest among pediatricians.[1,2] Febrile illnesses are frequent in infancy. In fact, in each of the first three years of life, children in day care have seven to nine respiratory illnesses, about one-third of which are accompanied by fever.[3] Most episodes are minor and usually resolve without use of antimicrobial agents. A number of febrile illnesses have an identifiable focus such as acute otitis media. But in approximately 3% to 10% of febrile infants, invasive bacterial infection is present and may be documented by a culture of blood.[4] The bacteremia is usually unanticipated and thus has been termed "occult bacteremia."

The children most likely to have occult bacteremia are less than 24 months of age with temperature $\geq 103^{o}$F and white blood cell counts in excess of 15,000 per ml (or some other laboratory indication of inflammatory reaction such as elevated sedimentation rate or presence of C-reactive proteins). About one-third of children with occult bacteremia recover without antibiotics, meaning that the bacteremia clears and the clinical signs resolve within 24 to 72 hours. However, most of the other children do not improve, and some develop severe or focal disease if appropriate antimicrobial therapy is not instituted.[5-7] Occult bacteremia progressed to meningitis in 4% of children with pneumococcal bacteremia,[5] 7% of children with bacteremia due to *Hemophilus influenzae*[6] and 25% of a group with occult meningococcemia.[7]

Use of antimicrobial agents for the child with risk features of occult bacteremia has been controversial. Results of investigations at Boston City Hospital,[5,6] Michael Reese Hospital[8] and Children's Hospital of Cincinnati[9] suggest that children who have bacteremia and are treated as outpatients with an antimicrobial agent have a better outcome than children who are not treated. In contrast, usage of amoxicillin in a large randomized trial conducted in Philadelphia and Chicago failed to show benefit of the antimicrobial regimen.[10]

Experience with ceftriaxone for treatment of serious infections in infants and children including sepsis and meningitis has indicated efficacy and safety in a once or twice a day dosage schedule.[11-13] Ceftriaxone is a parenteral third-generation cephalosporin with *in vitro* efficacy against *Streptococcus pneumoniae*, group A *Streptococci*, *Staphylococcus aureus*, *H. influenzae*, *Neisseria meningitidis* and some gram-negative enteric bacilli. Ceftriaxone has characteristics that make it attractive for use in febrile children with presumed occult bacteremia. Its long half-life of approximately 6.5 to 8 hours provides effective serum and tissue concentrations for 24 hours; its spectrum of activity includes the major pathogens responsible for occult bacteremia (*S. pneumoniae*, *N. meningitidis* and *H. influenzae* type b).[11,12] Clinical trials suggest efficacy of a once-daily dosing schedule for serious infections including sepsis and meningitis in infants and children.[12,13]

Therefore, while a multicenter randomized trial of parenteral ceftriaxone or oral amoxicillin for treatment of infants with risk features of occult bacteremia is in progress, the characteristics of ceftriaxone warrant consideration of its use for children with presumed occult bacteremia who are treated outside the hospital.

Also, while for the present, use of antimicrobial agents for infants with risk features of occult bacteremia remains a matter of clinical judgment, it is unlikely that we will soon have better information until the multicenter trial of ceftriaxone is concluded. Despite the lack of conclusive evidence to show that antimicrobial therapy is beneficial for children with occult bacteremia, physicians are justified in choosing an antibiotic regimen for selected children with clinical features suggestive of bacteremia. Notably ceftriaxone has characteristics that make it a drug of potential benefit for these children.

ORAL REGIMENS FOR OTITIS MEDIA

Acute Illness

With appropriate antimicrobial therapy, most children with acute otitis media are significantly improved within 48 to 72 hours. Amoxicillin remains the preferred drug for initial therapy of acute otitis media. If the patient does not respond to initial therapy with amoxicillin, infection with a resistant strain of *H. influenzae* or *Branhamella catarrhalis* should be considered. If the child is toxic the physician may consider tympanocentesis to identify the causative organism; a specific antimicrobial agent may then be chosen on the basis of results of the culture of the middle ear effusion and sensitivity testing. If acute signs of ear disease persist but the child is not toxic, the initial antimicrobial regimen should be changed to take into account a resistant strain.

The problem of antibiotic resistance among strains of bacteria causing otitis media must be considered by the physician. Non-typable strains of *H. influenzae* are isolated from 20% to 30% of episodes of acute otitis media, and 20% to 30% of these strains are resistant to amoxicillin. Thus, 4% to 9% of all cases of otitis media are due to beta-lactamase producing strains of *H. influenzae*. The occurrence of *B. catarrhalis* as an important cause of otitis media is variable from community to community. A good generalization would be that 10% of episodes of otitis are due to *B. catarrhalis* and two-thirds of strains produce beta-lactamase and would be resistant to ampicillin or amoxicillin. Adding the proportion of otitis media due to beta-lactamase producing *H. influenzae* and *B. catarrhalis*, it is anticipated that 10% to 15% of strains of bacteria causing acute otitis media are resistant to amoxicillin.

It should, however, be noted that approximately one-third of the cases of bacterial otitis media clear without use of antimicrobial agents,[14] presumably because of evacuation of the middle ear abscess by drainage through the eustachian tube or by spontaneous perforation of the tympanic membrane. Thus, beta-lactamase producing *H. influenzae* or *B. catarrhalis* would be of clinical importance in 7% to 10% of cases of acute otitis media. Since the vast majority of children are likely to be treated effectively by amoxicillin with its 25 year record of safety and efficacy,[14] lower cost and acceptability by children, I continue to recommend amoxicillin as the preferred drug for initial treatment of acute otitis media. Investigators will continue to monitor susceptibility patterns of the bacterial pathogens of otitis media to determine if this recommendation will need to be reconsidered. Other regimens that are satisfactory include amoxicillin-clavulanate,[16] trimethoprim-sulfamethoxazole, erythromycin-sulfisoxazole, cefuroxime axetil, cefixime and cefaclor. No clinical or microbiologic differences have been noted in the efficacy of the various regimens for treatment of acute otitis media due to susceptible strains.

Notably, the value of ampicillin and amoxicillin for treatment of respiratory infections is limited by the resistance of bacteria that produce the enzyme beta-lactamase including *S. aureus*, non-typable and *H. influenzae* type b, *B. catarrhalis* and gram-negative bacilli.[16] Clavulanic acid has a nuclear structure similar to that of penicillin without an acylamino side-chain. Although it has no significant anti-bacterial activity, clavulanic acid acts as an irreversible inhibitor of beta-lactamase.[16] Clavulanic acid binds to the active site of the beta-lactamase resulting in the formation of a stable and inactive clavulanic-beta-lactamase complex. Thus, amoxicillin-clavulanate broadens the spectrum of activity of the active drug, amoxicillin, to include previously resistant beta-lactamase producing strains.

Otitis Media with Effusion

Fluid usually persists in the middle ear of children for weeks to months after each episode of acute otitis media.[17] A conductive hearing loss (median loss is 25 decibels) is present whenever fluid fills the middle ear. Because of concern that impairment of hearing during infancy may affect development of speech, language and cognitive abilities, pediatricians have sought medical and surgical therapies for ridding the middle ear of fluid. Ventilating tubes that drain middle ear fluid and allow for aeration of the middle ear and recovery of the health of the middle ear mucosa have become the second most frequently performed surgical procedure in infants and children (exceeded in number only by circumcision).[17]

The results of studies to identify a medical regimen to clear middle ear fluid that follows acute otitis media have met with limited success. Decongestants and antihistamines are of little value. Steroids have been effective in some children, but insufficient follow-up leaves the benefit of the therapy unresolved. Pathogenic bacteria are present in approximately one-third of ears at the time of placement of ventilating tubes. Studies of use of trimethoprim-sulfamethoxazole and cefaclor have indicated some value of antimicrobial agents in resolution of otitis media with effusion.[18] The most compelling data for efficacy of an antibiotic regimen to decrease time spent with middle ear effusion was provided by Mandel and colleagues.[19] The rate of resolution of middle ear effusion was twice as high in children treated with amoxicillin as those who were treated with placebo. These data are sufficiently compelling to suggest that a trial of two weeks of an antimicrobial agent having a spectrum of activity to include all possible pathogens, including beta-lactamase producing strains, should be instituted before the child has a procedure for placement of ventilating tubes. Amoxicillin-clavulanate, trimethoprim-sulfamethoxazole, erythromycin-sulfisoxazole or cefaclor would be appropriate in a therapeutic dosage schedule. If, at the end of the two-week course the effusion persists, an operative procedure should be performed.

Prevention of Recurrences of Acute Otitis Media

As noted, acute otitis media is one of the most common infectious diseases of childhood. By three years of age approximately two-thirds of children have had at least one episode of acute otitis media and one-third of children have had three or more episodes.[20] Some children have six or more acute illnesses.[20] The results of ten clinical trials indicate that children at risk for recurrent episodes of acute otitis media who received a prophylactic antibiotic regimen had fewer episodes of acute infection than did untreated children.[21] The decrease in new episodes varied between 60% and 90%.

Most studies used a sulfonamide, usually sulfisoxazole, or a penicillin such as amoxicillin. Adverse effects of the antimicrobial agents were similar to those identified for therapeutic courses including mild gastrointestinal upset and rash. No reports of an increased incidence of serious reactions due to prolonged usage of these drugs has appeared. Importantly, there has been no significant increase in resistance to respiratory bacteria in patients receiving prolonged courses for prophylaxis.

Based on the results of the clinical trials, the following prophylactic program was suggested in 1982:[21]

• *Criteria for enrollment:* Three episodes of acute otitis media in six months or four episodes in one year.

• *Choice of antimicrobial agent:* Amoxicillin or sulfisoxazole.

• *Dosage schedule:* Half the therapeutic dose administered once-a-day, preferably at a time that would increase compliance, i.e., at breakfast or at bedtime, amoxicillin in a dose equal to 20 mg/kg/day or sulfisoxazole in a dose equal to 50 mg/kg/day.

• *Duration:* Up to six months or during the period of high incidence of infections of the respiratory tract in winter or spring.

• *Treatment of acute otitis media during prophylaxis:* Choose the alternative agent in a therapeutic dosage schedule (if amoxicillin was used for prophylaxis, use trimethoprim-sulfamethoxazole or erythromycin-sulfisoxazole or cefaclor or cefixime or cefuroxime axetil; if sulfisoxazole was used for prophylaxis use amoxicillin, amoxicillin-clavulanate or cefaclor or cefixime or cefuroxime axetil). After therapy, the prophylactic regimen is resumed.

• *If recurrences reappear after cessation of prophylaxis the prophylactic regimen should be restarted.*

• *Observation during prophylaxis:* The prophylactic regimen may not affect the appearance or persistence of asymptomatic middle ear effusion; therefore, children should be followed at four-to-six week intervals to determine if management of fluid in the middle ear is required.

MANAGEMENT OF CONTACTS OF PATIENTS WITH INVASIVE DISEASE DUE TO *H. INFLUENZAE* TYPE B OR *N. MENINGITIDIS*

Care of Contacts of Patients with Invasive Disease Due to *H. influenzae*

Secondary or concurrent cases of disease due to *H. influenzae* are of particular concern in infants under four years of age. Asymptomatic carriage is high in household contacts of patients with disease due to this organism. Rifampin eradicates *H. influenzae* from the upper respiratory tract in most carriers, and data from the Centers for Disease Control in Atlanta suggest that use of rifampin reduces the incidence of invasive illness in exposed household contacts. Although chemoprophylaxis for contacts under four years of age has been practiced for almost 20 years, changes of recommendations by authoritative groups such as the Committee on Infectious Diseases of the American Academy of Pediatrics have created some confusion.

The following recommendations are those of the author but are also compatible with the 1988 edition of the Report of the Committee on Infectious Diseases (the Redbook) of the American Academy of Pediatrics:[22]

- *Careful observation of infants 48 months of age and younger:* Since disease may be concurrent with, as well as secondary to the index case, careful observation is essential. Parents should be informed that during the two weeks following exposure febrile illnesses should be reported to the physician at once.
- *Household contacts:* Rifampin prophylaxis is recommended for adults and children in those households with at least one contact younger than 48 months. Prior immunization of infants with *H. influenzae* type b polysaccharide vaccine does not alter this recommendation.
- *Day care and nursery school:* The advisability of rifampin prophylaxis in day care contacts is controversial. This author believes that following diagnosis of a case of invasive disease due to *H. influenzae* type b in day care centers with children under four years of age all children and adult caretakers should receive prophylaxis with rifampin.

The Red Book distinguishes between day care where there is prolonged contact and day care with limited contact. Prophylaxis is recommended for day care homes resembling households, such as those with children in which contact is 25 hours per week or more. The Committee does not recommend prophylaxis in day care facilities where all contacts are more than two years of age. The Committee does advise administering rifampin to all attendees and supervisory personnel when two or more cases of invasive disease have occurred among attendees within 60 days.

- *Index cases:* The patient may continue to harbor *H. influenzae* in the mucosa of the upper respiratory tract even though the disease has been adequately treated and the pathogen eliminated from body fluids and tissues. Since the organism may be reintroduced into the household by the index case, the patient who is returning to households with contacts 48 months or younger should also receive prophylaxis before discharge from the hospital.

• *Pregnant women:* The effects of rifampin on the fetus are still uncertain; therefore, pregnant women should not receive the drug for prophylaxis.

• *Dosage schedules:* Rifampin is administered by mouth once daily for four days in a dosage of 20 mg/kg/dose (maximum dose is 600 mg).

Care of Contacts of Patients with Invasive Disease Due to *N. meningitidis*

Less controversy and little change has occurred in recommendations for prophylaxis of contacts of patients with meningococcal disease.[23] Observation of exposed household, school or day care contacts is an important part of any plan once a case has been identified. Rifampin prophylaxis is warranted for adult and child contacts of the index case in the household, day care center or nursery school. Sulfisoxazole is considered for prophylaxis only when an isolate is known to be susceptible.

• *Dosage schedule:* Rifampin at 10 mg/kg/dose (maximum 600 mg) every 12 hours for a total of four doses or sulfisoxazole for two days at 500 mg once daily for infants less than one year, 500 mg every 12 hours for children 1 to 12 years, and 1 gm every 12 hours for children more than 12 years of age and adults.

• *Meningococcal vaccine:* Because cases may occur in contacts weeks after the index case, the quadrivalent meningococcal vaccine should be used in contacts. For infants under 18 months of age, only group A meningococcal component of the vaccine is effective. Group C (and presumably Y and W-135) are effective only in children two years of age and older.

Of note, a single dose of a quinolone, ciprofloxacin, was effective in eliminating chronic nasopharyngeal carriage of *N. meningitidis* suggesting an effective mode of prophylaxis for contacts of cases of invasive disease due to this organism.[24,25]

The Quinolones

The quinolones are structurally related to nalidixic acid which has been in use since 1962. The drugs are currently available in oral forms, but parenteral preparations are under investigation. The quinolones have a broad spectrum of activity including many difficult-to-treat respiratory pathogens such as *Pseudomonas aeruginosa*, beta-lactamase producing *H. influenzae*, methicillin-resistant *S. aureus*, and *Chlamydia trachomatis*. Quinolones, currently approved by the FDA for marketing in the United States, include ciprofloxacin and norfloxacin. Of note, it has been observed that the quinolones accumulate in cartilage, and blister formation and ulcerations have been observed in cartilage of young experimental animals, mainly in weight-bearing joints.[26] Although these data are difficult to extrapolate to man, the animal data are of sufficient concern to warrant contraindication for usage in children through adolescence. Although not to be used in children, the drugs are of sufficient interest so that pediatricians need to be aware of the pharmacology and clinical usage of the quinolones. The potential benefit of an oral agent with efficacy against *P. aeruginosa* and *S. aureus* suggests value for patients with cystic fibrosis. Usage of ciprofloxacin in 150 adult patients with cystic fibrosis was discussed at a recent workshop in Edinburgh.[27] The proceedings of a symposium about clinical and pharmacologic data about new quinolones are presented in two issues of the Review of Infectious Diseases.[28,29]

It is possible that sometime in the future, sufficient experience about safety and efficacy of the quinolones will be available from humane usage in children who are critically ill with organisms uniquely susceptible, to warrant reconsideration of pediatric usage.

Reappearance of Rheumatogenic Strains of Group A Streptococci

During the past few years an increase in incidence of rheumatic fever has been identified in the United States, specifically in Salt Lake City,[30] Akron[31] and Pittsburgh.[32] In addition, a major increase in rheumatic fever occurred among recruits at the San Diego Naval Station. Streptococci isolated during epidemics are generally rich in M protein and richly encapsulated; strains associated with sporadic group A streptococcal pharyngitis lack capsules and are low in M protein. Both M protein and the hyaluronic acid are associated with increased virulence and rheumatogenicity. A factor in the apparent resurgence of acute rheumatic fever may be the reappearance of group A streptococci with enhanced rheumatogenic potential, which are mucoid strains resistant to phagocytosis because of the presence of large amounts of surface M protein.[33] Bacteriologic surveys carried out in Salt Lake City, Utah and in Columbus, Ohio during the period of increased incidence of rheumatic fever revealed the presence of highly mucoid streptococcal strains of M types 3 and 18,[34] Only time and careful surveillance will reveal whether we are at the beginning of a period of renewed incidence and severity of infection due to group A streptococci or are only witnessing a transient increase in a continually declining incidence curve of acute rheumatic fever. The reappearance of a heretofore relatively rare streptococcal serotype (M18) in multiple areas of the United States and its association with acute rheumatic fever outbreaks provides support to the hypothesis that rheumatogenic strains of group A streptococci exist.[34]

EMERGENCE OF ANTIBIOTIC RESISTANCE

Streptococcus pneumoniae

Multiresistant strains of *S. pneumoniae* that are highly resistant to penicillin G (minimum inhibitory concentration [MIC] more than 4 mcg/ml) were first noted in South Africa in 1977[35] and have remained restricted to that area. Few of these strains have been identified in the United States and Western Europe. However, many strains of *S. pneumoniae* that have been isolated in recent years have had decreased susceptibility to penicillin G (MIC 0.1 to 1.0 mcg/ml).

Haemophilus influenzae

Fifteen percent to 30% of both nontypable and type b strains of *H. influenzae* produce a beta-lactamase that hydrolyzes amoxicillin and penicillin G and V. The proportion of beta-lactamase producing strains has increased since such strains were first detected in 1974, but the proportion of these strains appears to be stabilizing in recent years. Regional differences and differences in time make any survey over a short period in a local area of uncertain significance for the overall pattern in the United States.

Resistance of *H. influenzae* to chloramphenicol remains rare, but occasional strains of combined ampicillin chloramphenicol resistance have been reported in the

United States and are of importance in Barcelona.[36] Physicians should be alert to changes in resistance patterns in their community.

Branhamella catarrhalis

Prior to 1971 almost all strains of *B. catarrhalis* were sensitive to penicillin and ampicillin. Today, in Western Europe and the United States a majority of strains, varying between 50% and 75% in various surveys, produce beta-lactamase. If the incidence of disease due to *B. catarrhalis* increases (as may occur in otitis media), usage of active drugs that are not altered by beta-lactamase will be needed for initial therapy.

Staphylococcus aureus and *Staphylococcus epidermidis*

For more than 30 years we have recognized that about one-third of strains of *S. aureus* from the community and the majority of strains in hospitals produce beta-lactamase. A small number of community strains (approximately 1%) but a significant number of hospital strains (particularly in small closed areas such as intensive care units) are resistant to the penicillinase-resistant penicillins (termed methicillin-resistant strains or MRSA) and require special attention when therapy of such a strain is needed. Most MRSA are sensitive to vancomycin or ciprofloxacin and to other selected antimicrobial agents.

S. epidermidis has become a pathogen of concern among hospitalized patients with intravascular or prosthetic devices. Most strains produce beta-lactamase. The incidence of methicillin resistance is higher for *S. epidermidis* than it is for *S. aureus.* Initial therapy for disease that may be caused by *S. epidermidis* must be considered carefully. Vancomycin or gentamicin may be used and the initial choice re-evaluated when results of susceptibility tests are available. Removal of the prosthetic device is often necessary to effect a cure.

Gram-negative bacilli: The choice of antibiotics for infections due to gram-negative bacteria depends on the particular pattern of susceptibility in the hospital or area of the patient. These patterns vary in different hospitals or communities and from time to time within the same institution. Susceptibility of gram-negative bacilli should be monitored to determine the emergence of new strains with unique antimicrobial susceptibility.

Group A Streptococci: No strains of group A streptococci resistant to penicillin G have been reported, but erythromycin resistant strains do occur.

Neisseria meningitidis: Dillon and colleagues[37] in 1983 reported isolation of a strain of *N. meningitidis* which contained the same type of beta-lactamase producing plasmid that has been isolated from *N. gonorrhoeae.*[29] This isolate probably originated in the genital tract and demonstrates the spread of antibiotic resistant plasmids among *Neisseria* species. This first isolation of a strain of a beta-lactamase producing *N. meningitidis* necessitates careful surveillance to determine the spread of such strains and the possible need to modify initial therapy of presumed meningococcal disease.

REFERENCES

1. The Febrile Infant and Occult Bacteremia. The Report of the Nineteenth Ross Roundtable; 1988 Ross Laboratories, Columbus, Ohio.
2. Klein JO. The febrile child and occult bacteremia. N Engl J Med 1987;317:1219-20.
3. Loda FA, Glezen WB, Clyde WA Jr. Respiratory disease in group day care. Pediatrics 1972;49:428-37.
4. Teele DW, Marshall R, Klein JO. Unsuspected bacteremia in young children. Pediatr Clin North Am 1979; 26:773-84.
5. Bratton L, Teele DW, Klein JO. Outcome of unsuspected pneumococcemia in children not initially admitted to hospital. J Pediatr 1977;90:703-6.
6. Marshall R, Teele DW, Klein JO. Unsuspected bacteremia due to *Haemophilus influenzae*: outcome in children not initally admitted to hospital. J Pediatr 1979;95:690-5.
7. Dashefsky B, Teele DW, Klein JO. Unsuspected meningococcemia. J Pediatr 1983;102:69-72.
8. Dershewitz RA, Wigder HN, Wigder CM, et al. A comparative study of the prevalence, outcome, and prediction of bacteremia in children. J Pediatr 1983;103:352-8.
9. Carroll WL, Farrell MK, Singer JI, et al. Treatment of occult bacteremia: a prospective randomized clinical trial. Pediatrics 1983;72:608-12.
10. Jaffe DW, Tanz RR, Davis AT, et al. Antibiotic administration to treat possible occult bacteremia in febrile children. N Engl J Med 1987; 317:1175-1180.
11. Word BW, Klein JO. Current therapy of bacterial sepsis and meningitis in infants and children: a poll of directors of programs in pediatric infectious diseases. Pediatr Infect Dis 1988;7:267-70.
12. Frenkel LD, and the Multicenter Ceftriaxone Pediatric Study Group. Once-daily administration of ceftriaxone for the treatment of selected serious bacterial infections in children. Pediatrics 1988;82:486-91.
13. Yogev R, Shulman ST, Chadwick EG, et al. Once daily ceftriaxone for central nervous system infections and other serious pediatric infections. Pediatr Infect Dis 1986;5:298-303.
14. Halstead C, Lepow M, Balassanian N, et al. Otitis media: clinical observation, microbiology and evaluation of therapy. Am J Dis Child 1968;115:542-51.
15. Odio CM, Kusniesz RM, Shelton S, et al. Comparative treatment trial of augmentin vs. cefaclor for acute otitis media with effusion. Pediatrics 1985;75:819-26.
16. Bush K. Recent developments in B-lactamase research and their implications for the future. Rev Infect Dis 1988;10:681-90.
17. Bluestone CD, Klein JO. In: Otitis Media in Infants and Children. Philadelphia: W.B. Saunders Co., 1988:132-65.
18. Healy GB. Antimicrobial therapy of chronic otitis media with effusion. J Infect Pediatr Otorhinolaryngol 1984;8:13-7.
19. Mandell EM, Rockett HE, Bluestone CD, et al. Efficacy of amoxicillin with and without decongestant-antihistamine for otitis media with effusion in children: results of a double-blind, randomized trial. N Engl J Med 1987;316:432-7.
20. Teele Dw, Klein JO, Rosner B, et al. Epidemiology of otitis media during the first seven years of life in children in greater Boston: a prospective, cohort study. J Infect Dis 1989;160:83-94.
21. Klein JO, Bluestone CD. Acute otitis media. Pediatr Infect Dis 1982;1:66-73.
22. American Academy of Pediatrics. *Hemophilus influenzae* infections: control measures. In: Peter G, ed. Report of the committee of infectious diseases. 20th ed., Elk Grove Village, IL: American Academy of Pediatrics, 1988:203-4.

23. American Academy of Pediatrics. Meningococcal infections: control measures. In: Peter G, ed. Report of the committee of infectious diseases. 20th ed., Elk Grove Village, IL: American Academy of Pediatrics, 1988:286-8.
24. Pugsley MP, Dworzack DL, Roccaforte JS, et al. An open study of the efficacy of a single dose of ciprofloxacin in eliminating the chronic nasopharyngeal carriage of *Neisseria meningitidis*. J Infect Dis 1988;157:852-3.
25. Gaunt PN. Ciprofloxacin vs ceftriaxone for eradication of meningococcal carriage. Lancet 1988;218-9.
26. Christ W, Lehnert T, Ulbrick B. Specific toxicologic aspects of the quinolones. Rev Infect Dis 1988;10:141S-146S.
27. Raeburn JA, Govan JRW, McCrae WM, et al. Ciprofloxacin therapy in cystic fibrosis. J Antimicrob Chemother 1987; 20:295-6.
28. Rubinstein E, Adam D, Moellering R, et al. IInternational symposium on new quinolones. Rev Infect Dis 1988;10:1S-271S.
29. Rubinstein E, Adam D, Moellering R, et al. Second international symposium on the new quinolones. Rev Infect Dis 1989;11:897S-1431S.
30. Veasy LG, Wiedmeier SE, Orsmond GS, et al. Resurgence of acute rheumatic fever in the intermountain area of the United States. N Engl J Med 1987; 316:421-7.
31. Cogneni B, Rizzo C, Congeni J, et al. Outbreak of acute rheumatic fever in northeast Ohio. J Pediatr 1987; 111:176-9.
32. Wald ER, Dashefsky B, Feidt C, et al. Acute rheumatic fever in western Pennsylvania and the tristate area. Pediatrics 1987;80:371-4.
33. Kaplan EL, Hill HR. Return of rheumatic fever: consequences, implications and needs. J Pediatr 1987;111:244-6.
34. Marcon MJ, Hribar MM, Hosier DM, et al. Occurrence of mucoid M-18 *Streptococcus pyogenes* in a central Ohio pediatric population. J Clin Microbiol 1988;26:1539-42.
35. Applebaum PC, Bhamjee A, Scragg JN, et al. *Streptococcus pneumoniae* resistant to penicillin and chloramphenicol. Lancet 1977;2:955-97.
36. Marques JC, Garcia-Tornel S, Tahull JMG. Invasive infections caused by multiply resistant *Haemophilus influenzae* type b. J Pediatr 1984;104:162.
37. Dillon JR, Pauze M, Yeung K-H. Spread of penicillinase-producing and transfer plasmids from the gonococcus to *Neisseria meningitidis*. Lancet 1983;1:779-80.

CHAPTER 9

Outpatient Management of Lower Respiratory Tract Infection

Louis D. Saravolatz, M.D.
Detroit, Michigan

INTRODUCTION

The topic of lower respiratory tract infection is usually discussed in relation to the site of acquisition (i.e., community or hospital acquired), the extent of infection (i.e., tracheobronchitis or pneumonia) and the etiologic agents. Within each of these classifications, the physician may consider outpatient versus inpatient management, and there are multiple factors that play a role in determining whether hospitalization is necessary. These include host factors, severity of illness, patient compliance, economic considerations and social factors. This chapter will review the epidemiology, microbiology, clinical manifestations and therapy of lower respiratory tract infections in the *normal host*, with emphasis on community-acquired disease or hospital acquired pneumonia for which therapy may be completed as an outpatient.

EPIDEMIOLOGY

Respiratory infections are common in the outpatient setting. In a prospective study of 292 individuals evaluated between 1948 and 1950 in Cleveland, Dingle identified 4428 respiratory infections, of which there were 29 patients with atypical pneumonia and only three cases of pneumococcal pneumonia.[1] If we extrapolate from the Dingle study, we can estimate that there are 2.5 million to 4 million cases of atypical pneumonia per year, most of which would be cared for in the ambulatory setting. Also, it is estimated that there are 150,000 to 570,000 cases of pneumococcal pneumonia per year.[2]

Of note, the risk of pneumonia is clearly increased in patients who are immunosuppressed with malignancy or who have recently undergone organ transplantation.[3,4,5] In addition, there are specific host defects that predispose patients to develop pneumonia, which include endotracheal intubation, tracheostomy, IgA deficiency, defects in the mucociliary apparatus, acquired hypogammaglobulinemia (IgG_2 and IgG_4), and C_3 and C_5 deficiency. Other risk factors known to be associated with the development of pneumonia include the extremes of age, alcohol abuse, chronic lung disease, smoking and recent viral respiratory infection.

PATHOGENESIS

Although oropharyngeal aspiration occurs with some regularity, lower respiratory tract infection is not a regular sequelae.[3] Indeed, normal host defense mechanisms prevent the inoculum of aspirated pathogenic organisms from causing lower respiratory tract infections. However, if the normal defense mechanisms are overwhelmed or impaired when the host aspirates, pneumonia may result. In order for bacterial pneumonia to occur, the host must first be colonized with pathogenic bacteria. The scenario of colonization with pathogenic bacteria and the subsequent development of aspiration pneumonia can occur in the community or hospital setting. The factors that regulate the bacterial flora of the upper respiratory tract have been intensively studied over the past few years.[6] A variety of factors have been suggested as being important in the selection of colonizing pathogenic organisms, including ph, redox potential, temperature, nutrient supply, lysozyme and bacteriocins.[6] However, when considering the great variety of bacterial species that coexist in the oropharynx, these factors are felt to exert a relatively weak influence on colonization.

ADHERENCE

Adherence, the relative ability of bacterial species to attach to epithelial cells, is an important factor in bacterial colonization. Secretory immunoglobulin (IgA) may coat some bacterial species and prevent adherence. Cell surfaces of buccal epithelial cells play an important role in *cell-cell* recognition and adhesion. These *cell-cell* surface interactions permit a preferential adherence of certain bacteria over other bacteria.[7] Studies have demonstrated that in patients colonized with gram-negative bacilli, buccal epithelial cells had greater adherence than in non-colonized patients. Moreover, specific alteration of fibronectin on the surface of epithelial cells permits adherence of gram-negative bacilli.[8]

COLONIZATION

In general, colonization with gram-negative bacilli does not regularly occur. The prevalence of gram-negative bacilli within the oropharynx ranges between 2% and 18%.[9,10] However, in a study by Valenti and colleagues, gram-negative colonization was evaluated in elderly individuals, and it was found that in those over the age of 65, colonization occurred in 3% to 60% of those tested.[11] Colonization was greater in patients who had a decrease in their level of activity. In the Valenti study, 3% of ambulatory hospital volunteers were colonized, 9% of patients in senior citizens, apartments were colonized, 22% of patients in nursing homes were colonized and 60% of bedridden patients in the hospital were colonized. The risk factors associated with colonization included underlying cardiac, pulmonary and neoplastic disorders, bladder incontinence and bedridden clinical status. The gram-negative bacilli found by Valenti included *Klebsiella pneumoniae* (41%), *Escherichia coli* (24%), *Enterobacter sp.* (14%), *Pseudomonas aeruginosa* (5%) and *Proteus mirabilis* (4%).

MECHANISMS

Bacterial pneumonia can occur by one of four mechanisms: (1) aspiration; (2) inhalation of aerosols; (3) hematogenous seeding; and (4) contiguous spread. Aspiration is the most common mechanism and occurs following colonization with pathogenic organisms. Aspiration of oral flora was studied by Amberson in 1937.[12]

A more recent study by Huxley in 1978 confirmed some of the original observations.[13] In particular, the study demonstrated that aspiration during sleep is a normal physiologic event both in healthy individuals and in patients with neurologic impairment. In the study, two groups of subjects were evaluated for the occurrence of aspiration during normal sleep.[13] Subjects had a nasopharyngeal catheter placed and radioactive contrast material injected after they had fallen asleep. The following day, lung scanning was performed to see where the contrast material had lodged. One of the groups of subjects was comprised of healthy volunteers who were observed to aspirate 45% of the time while sleeping. The second group of subjects included patients with neurologic impairment, and in this group aspiration occurred in 70% of the subjects. Also, aspiration was more likely to occur when the patients reached a deeper level of sleep.

MICROBIOLOGY

Sullivan reviewed 292 cases of community-acquired pneumonia and found 41 patients (23%) with serologically confirmed viral pneumonia among the 175 patients who had complete serologic tests.[14] The viral agents identified included influenza, parainfluenza, and adenovirus. Also, the Sullivan study described the bacterial etiology in 167 cases of community-acquired pneumonia. The distribution of bacterial pathogens was *Streptococcus pneumoniae* (62%); gram-negative bacilli, (20%); *Staphylococcus aureus* (10%); and *Hemophilus influenzae* (8%). In other series of community-acquired pneumonia, *S. pneumoniae* has accounted for 65% to 94% of bacterial isolates.[15,16] The role of mycoplasma in studies of community-acquired pneumonia is probably underrepresented. Patients included in such studies usually require hospitalization, whereas most patients with *Mycoplasma pneumoniae* pneumonia respond to outpatient therapy and seldom require hospitalization. In addition, not all patients studied have had serologic tests performed for mycoplasma.

M. pneumoniae has been implicated in 11% to 17% of pneumonia in patients over 40 years of age.[17]

Chlamydial pneumonia may be caused by *Chlamydia psittaci* or *Chlamydia trachomatis*. Although these agents are relatively uncommon in the adult, there have been recent reports of healthy adults developing community-acquired pneumonia due to the chlamydia - TWAR strain.[18,19]

Legionella pneumophila appears to be a common cause of community or hospital acquired pneumonia. The frequency of this problem varies with environmental exposure and host susceptibility. Nonetheless, there are some who feel legionella may occur in as many as 15% of community-acquired pneumonias.[20,21] However, a more representative estimation of the prevalence of legionella is probably 1% to 10%.[20,22]

CLINICAL MANIFESTATION

When presented with a patient with a lower respiratory tract infection, the clinician must review the history, physical examination, chest radiographs and laboratory findings to answer four questions: (1) *What is the most likely microbiologic etiology of the patient's infection?*; (2) *Is the infection an acute bronchitis or pneumonia?*; (3) *Does the severity of illness mandate hospitalization of the patient?*; (4) *What is the preferred therapy?*

A variety of clinical clues have been helpful in distinguishing the various etiologies of pneumonia. The most common pathogens are viruses and two bacteria, *S. pneumoniae*, and *M. pneumoniae*. If the patient has chronic lung disease, other pathogens may also play a role such as *H. influenzae, S. aureus, Branhamella catarrhalis*, or gram-negative enteric bacilli. If the host is debilitated, gram-negative organism, including legionella, may be important. In cystic fibrosis patients, *P. aeruqinosa* and *S. aureus* are the major pathogens.

The environmental setting for pneumonia may be important. *M. pneumoniae* is frequently acquired in school or in other close quarters where young people congregate. Legionella was originally implicated in certain hospitals, hotels or excavation sites. However, since the Philadelphia epidemic of 1976, we have learned that this organism is ubiquitous and may cause epidemic and non-epidemic pneumonia.

TABLE I. Clinical manifestations of *S. pneumoniae*, *M. pneumoniae*, and *L. pneumophila* (modified from Helms, et al in reference 23)

	S. pneumoniae	*M. pneumoniae*	*L. pneumophila*
Duration of symptoms before presentation	2-3 days	12 days	4-5 days
URI symptoms	50%	40%	0%
Cough	95%	100%	50%
Nausea/vomiting	30-40%	30-40%	30-40%
Diarrhea	5%	10%	20%
Fever	++	+	+++
Temperature-Pulse disparity	0	++	+++

Historical information may be helpful in suggesting an etiology of the lower respiratory tract infection (Table I.).[23] Patients with *M. pneumoniae* pneumonia may have symptoms for a prolonged period before seeking medical attention. These symptoms are suggestive of an upper respiratory tract illness and include rhinorrhea, cough, sore throat, headache and earache. *S. pneumoniae* patients may have similar symptoms, but are ill for a considerably shorter period of time (two to three days) before they seek medical attention. Legionella patients are often ill for several days, but have the absence of upper respiratory tract symptoms. Cough is usually not productive, if present. Although gastrointestinal symptoms have been suggested as more frequent with *L. pneumophila*, nausea and vomiting occur with equal frequency in cases of *S. pneumoniae* and *M. pneumoniae* pneumonia.[23]

Diarrhea, however, does occur with greater frequency in cases of legionella.[23] Of note, physical assessment is indistinguishable in pneumonia caused by *S. pneumoniae, M. pneumoniae*, or *L. pneumophila*, except for the presence of a temperature-pulse disparity, which does not occur in patients with *S. pneumoniae* unless they have a cardiac conduction defect or are receiving beta-blockers.

Laboratory tests have been suggested as being helpful in the diagnosis. Certainly, a white blood cell count of over 20,000/mm^3 is suggestive of a bacterial etiology. However, intermediate counts are frequently found and are not helpful. Chemistry abnormalities suggestive of legionella infection have included hyponatremia, hypophosphatemia or liver enzyme elevations. These tests, however, are non-specific in suggesting an etiology for pneumonia.

Chest radiographs will help define the presence and extent of the pneumonia. Pneumonia may be radiographically unapparent early in the course of the illness due to dehydration, leukopenia or minimal early involvement. Also, the clinician must distinguish pneumonia from other radiographic abnormalities caused by congestive heart failure, atelectasis, pulmonary embolism or other lung diseases. Once the diagnosis of pneumonia is made, the clinician needs to define the extent of disease and determine as to whether there is an accumulation of pleural fluid or whether an abscess is developing. Radiographic findings may suggest a need for hospitalization or an invasive procedure such as a thoracentesis.

Radiographic abnormalities of pneumonias have been suggested as diagnostic for certain etiologic agents. However, in my experience, there is extensive overlap in the radiographic abnormalities for various microbial pathogens, and specific etiologic agents cannot be diagnosed with a high degree of certainty from the chest X-ray.

DIAGNOSTIC CONSIDERATIONS

The sputum examination is a rapid, useful test that can be performed in the outpatient setting to assist the clinician in confirming an infection of the respiratory tract and in recognizing a specific etiologic agent. Cooperative, alert, adult patients should be instructed to provide lower respiratory tract secretions from a deep cough. This process can sometimes be assisted by chest percussion. Once obtained, the specimen should be Gram's stained for cytologic examination and description of the microbial morphology. The presence of large numbers (>25/low power field) of squamous epithelial cells that have exfoliated from the oropharyngeal cavity suggests that the specimen is contaminated with upper respiratory secretions. If there are <10 squamous epithelial cells/low power field, the correlation with transtracheal aspiration is good. If the sputum submitted demonstrates a large number of squamous epithelial cells, an additional specimen should be requested.

The Gram's stained smear may disclose a suggestive microbial morphology for organisms such as *S. pneumoniae, H. influenzae, S. aureus, B. catarrhalis*, or enteric bacilli. Sputum examination in patients with *M. pneumoniae* or acute purulent tracheobronchitis reveals a predominance of polymorphonuclear leukocytes (PMNs) without associated bacteria. In *L. pneumophila*, frequently no sputum is produced initially, and later several days into the illness, a Gram's stain will reveal PMNs without bacteria.

H. influenzae has been resistant to ampicillin in up to 22% of isolates at Henry Ford Hospital. If a physician encounters a high rate of ampicillin-resistant *H. influenzae* in his/her geographic area, then agents with activity against beta-lactamase producing strains should be selected. These agents include amoxicillin/clavulanic acid, cefuroxime and ciprofloxacin. If *S. aureus* is suspected, then one needs to select an agent resistant to beta-lactamase degradation. Thus, dicloxacillin, cephalosporins, amoxicillin/clavulanic, or clindamycin may be selected.

The selection of an oral antibiotic effective against gram-negative organisms in the outpatient setting limits the clinician to sulfamethoxazole/trimethoprim or ciprofloxacin. Sulfamethoxazole/trimethoprim is active against most gram-negative agents colonizing the respiratory tract, except for *P. aeruginosa*. In the case of *P. aeruginosa*, especially in cystic fibrosis patients, ciprofloxacin is the only oral agent available. Although another quinolone, norfloxacin, is available, its tissue penetration and low *in vitro* activity against *P. aeruginosa* prevent it from being considered in the treatment of respiratory tract infections. Other quinolones, enoxacin and ofloxacin, will be available in the near future but these agents appear to have less antipseudomonal activity than ciprofloxacin. In using ciprofloxacin for the treatment of *P. aeruginosa* acute tracheobronchitis, the clinician must limit therapy to two to three weeks. Therapy will select for resistance. With only three weeks of ciprofloxacin treatment, resistance rose from 8.3% (2/24 on day 1) to 69.6% (16/23 on day 21) of patients.[30] The MIC_{90} during the same interval rose from 0.5 mcg/ml to 8.0 mcg/ml.

In general, if gram-negative pneumonia is documented, hospitalization and parenteral therapy should be initiated to achieve a more rapid response. Once a satisfactory response has been achieved, then continuation of therapy in the outpatient setting with ciprofloxacin may be considered by the physician if the organism is susceptible and if the patient can tolerate oral medications.

In cases of anaerobic pneumonias, multiple pathogens are presumably responsible for causing the formation of a purulent lung abscess. These pathogens include *Fusobacterium necrophorum, Bacteroides melaninogenicus, Peptostreptococcus sp., Peptococcus sp.*, and microaerophilic streptococci. Studies have shown that 60% of *B. melaninogenicus* are penicillinase producers and are resistant to 2 mcg/ml of penicillin.[31] In a study of community-acquired putrid lung abscess, Levison and colleagues showed that clindamycin-treated patients had a shorter febrile period, fewer days of fetid sputum, fewer infectious complications and a higher cure rate than did patients treated with penicillin.[32] Clindamycin-treated patients were initially administered clindamycin 600 mg q 8 h intravenously for three to ten days, then switched to oral therapy with clindamycin at a dose of 300 mg q 6 h. However, clindamycin use still requires two notes of caution: (1) Clindamycin-resistant anaerobes have been reported, thus the longevity of clindamycin as a first-line anti-anaerobic agent could be limited; and (2) there needs to be an ongoing vigilance for the potential antibiotic-associated colitis that may be induced by clindamycin. Therefore, if diarrhea develops, clindamycin should be promptly discontinued and an evaluation for *C. difficile* toxin production performed.

A new oral cephalosporin, cefuroxime axetil, has recently been approved by the FDA for the treatment of lower respiratory tract infections. Its *in vitro* spectrum shows activity against *S. pneumoniae, H. influenzae,* and *B. catarrhalis.* However, while cefuroxime has potential as an alternative to amoxicillin, amoxcillin-clavulanic acid or sulfamethoxazole/trimethoprim, its high cost and limited clinical experience suggest limited and cautious use at this time. Also, although vaccines are not part of the management of the acute lower respiratory tract infections, they are important in preventing recurrences. Administration of pneumococcal vaccine should be considered in the high-risk pneumonia patient after the successful completion of therapy.

TABLE III. Drug interactions seen with antimicrobial agents prescribed for the outpatient management of lower respiratory tract infections

Antibiotic	Drug Interaction	Comment
Ampicillin	Allopurinol	Increased indication of skin rashes
	oral contraceptive	
		Decreased effectiveness of contraceptives
Erythromycin	Digitalis	Toxicity
	Theophylline	Toxicity
Ciprofloxacin	Theophylline	Toxicity
	Antacids	Decreased absorption (6-10X)
	Caffeine	Decreased caffeine clearance
Rifampin	Coumadin	Decreased anticoagulant effect
	Contraceptives	Decreased reliablity of contraception
	Corticosteroids	Decreased steroid effect
	Digitoxin	Decreased effect
	Methadone	Decreased effect
	Sulfonylureas	Hyperglycemia
Sulfamethoxazole/ trimethoprim	Coumadin	Enhanced anticoagulant effect
	Contraceptives	Decreased contraceptive effect
	Sulfonylureas	Hypoglycemia
	Phenytoin	Increased anticonvulsant effect
Tetracycline	Antacid	Decreased absorption
	Anticoagulant	Increased bleeding
	Bismuth subsalicylate	Decreased bioavailability
	Calcium supplements	Decreased absorption
	Colestipol	Decreased absorption
	Oral contraceptives	Decreased effectiveness of contraceptives
	Iron salts	Decreased absorption

In selecting an antimicrobial agent for pneumonia, the clinician must also consider potential drug interactions (Table III.). In particular, the clinician must be alert to the possibility of interactions of antibiotics with bronchodilators or other medications that are commonly administered for the illness. Erythromycin and ciprofloxacin both decrease the metabolism of theophylline and warrant serum theophylline level determinations. Another approach is to reduce the dose by one-third when starting these agents, but levels still need to be monitored.

The bioavailability of tetracycline and ciprofloxacin may be altered by divalent cations. Antacids, iron tablets and bismuth subsalicylate all decrease the absorption of tetracycline.[30] Thus, avoidance of these medications, or separating ingestion by at least two hours, is necessary. Only aluminum or magnesium containing antacids reduce absorption of ciprofloxacin. Therefore, either a calcium-containing antacid should be used with ciprofloxacin or a time interval should be required between ciprofloxacin ingestion and ingestion of antacids containing aluminum or magnesium.[33] Other important drug interactions between oral antibiotics and other medications are listed in Table III.[33]

TABLE IV. The cost of antimicrobial agents used in the outpatient management of lower respiratory tract infection*

Drug	Dose Frequency	Cost of 10 day course
Ampicillin	500 mg q6h	$ 9.44
Amoxicillin	500 mg q8h	12.80
Amoxicillin/ Clavulanic Acid	500 mg q8h	49.35
Cefuroxime axetil	500 mg q12h	72.83
Cephradine	500 mg q6h	36.08
Cephalexin	500 mg q6h	29.96
Ciprofloxacin	500 mg q12h	39.52
Ciprofloxacin	750 mg q12h	73.13
Clindamycin	300 mg q8h	58.74
Clindamycin	450 mg q8h	86.35
Dicloxacillin	500 mg q6h	28.00
Erythromycin	500 mg q6h	13.74
Doxycycline	100 mg q12h	8.49
Tetracycline	500 mg q6h	5.16
Sulfamethoxazole/ Trimethoprim	DS q12h	6.19
Rifampin	600 mg q12h	102.13

** Price based on 1988-89 Blue Book and a pharmacist average dispense fee ($3.50)*

When selecting an antibiotic for outpatient treatment of a lower respiratory tract infection, the clinican should select the least expensive agent that will meet the patient's needs. Of note, many of the newer agents are quite expensive and are not necessarily the preferred, or even an alternative agent (Table IV.).

FOLLOW-UP CARE

The physician should assure that the patient's clinical response is satisfactory. Subjective improvement should be encountered in three to five days with decreases in fever spikes, the amount of purulent sputum and other respiratory symptoms. A follow-up clinic visit should be scheduled for five to seven days after initiating antimicrobial chemotherapy. If no improvement is demonstrated or if clinical deterioration occurs before that visit, the patient should then be hospitalized. In summary, the patient's follow-up history and physical assessment are the most important means of evaluating the patient. A chest X-ray should only be considered if the patient is deteriorating. If the patient shows continued clinical improvement, a follow-up chest X-ray can be delayed until the completion of antimicrobial chemotherapy.

CONCLUSION

Lower respiratory tract infections continue to present a management challenge in the ambulatory setting. The physician must carefully assess the severity of the illness and determine whether hospitalization is necessary for optimal management. With current oral antimicrobial agents, most pathogens can be treated in an outpatient setting. However, delayed response, progession of the infection and the emergence of resistance may occur in the outpatient setting. To avoid or identify these problems early, the clinician must be prepared to closely monitor the patient's clinical response when treating lower respiratory tract infections in the ambulatory setting.

REFERENCES

1. Dingle JU, Badger GF, Feller AE, et al. A study of illness in a group of Cleveland families. Plan of study and certain general observations. Am J Hyg 1953;58:16-30.
2. Hoeprich PD. Bacterial pneumonias. In: Hoeprich PD, ed. Infectious diseases. Philadephia: Harper & Row, 1983:347-60.
3. Sanford JP. Lower respiratory tract infections. In: Bennet JV, Bachman PS, eds. Hospital infections. Boston: Little, Brown and Co., 1979:385-422.
4. LaForce FM. Hospital acquired gram negative rod pneumonias: an overview. Am J Med 1981;70:664-9.
5. Cross AS, Roup B. Role of respiratory assistance devices in endemic nosocomial pneumonia. Am J Med 1981;70:681-5.
6. Gibbons RJ, van Houte J. Bacterial adherence in oral microbial ecology. Ann Rev Microbiol 1975;29:1944.
7. Johanson WG Jr, Woods DE, Chaudhuri T. Association of respiratory tract colonization with adherence of gram-negative bacilli to epithelial cells. J Infect Dis 1979;139:667-73.
8. Woods DE, Straus DC, Johanson WG Jr, et al. Role of fibronectin in the prevention of adherence of *Pseudomonas aeruginosa* to buccal cells. J Infect Dis 1981;143 784-90.
9. Johanson WG, Pierce AK, Sanford JP. Changing pharyngeal bacterial flora in hospitalized patients - emergence of gram-negative bacilli. N Engl J Med 1969;281:1137-40.
10. Rosenthal S, Tager IB. Prevalence of gram-negative rods in the normal pharyngeal flora. Ann Intern Med 1975;83:355-7.
11. Valenti WM, Trudell RG, Bently DW. Factors predisposing to oropharyneal colonization with gram-negative bacilli in the aged. N Engl J Med 1978:298:1108-11.
12. Amberson JB. Aspiration bronchopneumonia. Int Clin 1937; 3:126.
13. Huxley EJ, Viroslav J, Gray WR, et al. Pharyngeal aspiration in normal adults and patients with depressed consciousness. Am J Med 1978;64:565.
14. Sullivan RJ, Dowdle WR, Marine WM, et al. Adult pneumonia in a general hospital. Arch Intern Med 1972;129:935-42.
15. Dorff GJ, Rytel MW, Farner SG, et al. Etiologies and characteristic features of pneumonia in a municipal hospital. Am J Med Sci 1973;266:349-50.
16. Fekety FR, Caldwell J, Gump D, et al. Bacteria, viruses, and mycoplasmas in acute pneumonia in adults. Am Rev Respir Dis 1971;104:499-507.

17. Murray HW, Maisur H, Senterfit LB, et al. The protein manifestations of *Mycoplasma pneumoniae* infection in adults. Am J Med 1975;58:229-42.
18. Grayston JT, Kuo CC, Wang SP, et al. A new chlamydia psittaci strain, TWAR, isolated from acute respiratory tract infections. N Engl J Med 1986;315:161-8.
19. Marrie TJ, Grayston T, Wang SP, et al. Pneumoniae associated with the TWAR strain of Chlamydia. Ann Intern Med 1987;106:507-11.
20. Balows A, Fraser DW (eds). International symposium on Legionnaires Disease. Ann Intern Med 1979;90:481-714.
21. MacFarlane JD, Finch RG, Wara MJ, et al. Hospital study of adult community aquired pneumonia. Lancet 1982; 2:255-8.
22. Foy HM, Broome CV, Hayes PS, et al. Legionnaires Disease in a prepaid medical-care group in Seattle 1963-75. Lancet 1979;1:767-70.
23. Helms CM, Viner JP, Sturn RH, et al. Comparative features of pneumococcal, mycoplasmal, and Legionnaires Disease pneumonia. Ann Intern Med 1979;90:543.
24. Steigbigel NH, Reed CW, Finland M. Susceptibility of common pathogenic bacterias to seven tetracycline antibiotics *in vitro*. Am J Med Sci 1968;255:179.
25. Glendinnen IJ. Doxycycline in the treatment of chronic lung infections. Med J Aust 1974;1:9.
26. Barber M, Waterworth PM. Penicillinase resistant penicillins and cephalosporins. Br Med J 1964;2:344.
27. Doern GV, Siebers KG, Halleik LM, et al. Antibiotic susceptibiltiy of beta-lactamase producing strains of Branhamella (Neisseria) catarrhalis. Antimicrob Agents Chemotherapy 1980;17:24.
28. McGehee RF, Smith CB, Wilcox F, et al. Comparative studies of antibacterial activity *in vitro* and absorption and excretion of lincomycin and clindamycin. Am J Med Sci 1968;256:279.
29. Kayser FH, Morak J. *In vitro* activity of ciprofloxacin as gram-positive bacteria. Am J Med 1987;82(4A):33-9.
30. Shalit I, Stutman H, Marks MI, et al. Randomized study of two dosage regimens of ciprofloxacin for treating chronic bronchopulmonary infection in patients with cystic fibrosis. Am J Med 1987;82(S4A):189-95.
31. Murray PR, Rosenblatt JE. Penicillin resistance and penicillinase production in clinical isolates of Bacteroides melaninogenicus. Antimicrob Agents Chemother 1977;11: 605-8.
32. Levison ME, Mangura CT, Lorber B, et al. Clindamycin compared with penicillin for the treatment of anaerobic lung abscess. Ann Intern Med 1983;98:466-71.

CHAPTER 10

Outpatient Antimicrobial Therapy of Acute Gastrointestinal Infections

Herbert L. DuPont, M.D.
Houston, Texas

INTRODUCTION

The most common clinical presentation of enteric infections is acute diarrhea. Diarrhea can be defined as an increase in stool frequency and a decrease in stool form when compared to the normal state. A more objective definition of diarrhea has been developed by gastrointestinal physiologists and physicians in charge of metabolic units, namely, the passage of more than 200 grams of stool per day with a decrease in stool form. Studies of the etiology of diarrhea have confirmed that most cases of acute illness are caused by definable pathogens. Many clinical and epidemiologic clues will help predict the cause likely to be present in a given patient.

DIAGNOSIS

Epidemiologic Association

A number of questions should be asked a patient with acute diarrhea to determine the setting in which the illness occurred. This will give valuable clues as to the proper work-up and ultimate management. A number of cases occurring in a given locale at the same time usually allows a diagnosis of a water-or food-borne illness acquisition. By establishing common exposure, it is often possible to establish an incubation period. Following determination of the incubation period, an evaluation of the most prevalent symptoms will usually determine the likely cause of the epidemic.

When travel precedes the illness, a special set of organisms appears likely; most infectious agents are acquired through the consumption of fecally contaminated food or water. The most common cause of acute diarrhea to travelers in developing countries are bacterial agents, of which enterotoxigenic *Escherichia coli* represents the most important single agent.[1] Toxigenic *E. coli* are usually culpable in cases acquired in South America, Africa, and Asia. On the other hand, when diarrhea occurs following travel to the Soviet Union, or to the mountainous regions of the United States and Canada, parasitic agents such as *Giardia* or *Cryptosporidia* should be suspected.

When illness occurs in a child who regularly attends a day care center or when symptoms occur in a teacher or even a parent of a child in a day care center, a special set of organisms should be considered. These include *Giardia*, *Cryptospordia*, *Shigella*, and rotavirus. Secondary spread into the family setting occurs commonly when an infant attending a day care center acquires illness.

Finally, homosexual males with diarrhea present a special diagnostic problem. These individuals acquire diarrhea either because of increased transmission of enteric organisms by fecal/oral route or because of the direct rectal inoculation of organisms during receptive anal intercourse. The high incidence of persistent diarrhea in AIDS or ARC represents a special problem which will not be discussed here.

Clinical Features

Diarrhea caused by infectious agents can vary in severity from slight to life-threatening. Bacterial, viral or protozoal pathogens may be implicated.

Fever: When evaluating patients with acute diarrhea, the physician should establish whether *fever* is a predominant feature of the disease. When fever is significant, the patient generally has an infection due to an invasive organism. The higher the fever and the more protracted the illness, the more likely the diarrhea is due to an invasive bacterial pathogen such as *Shigella, Salmonella,* or *Campylobacter.* Low grade fever is common with viral-induced enteric infection. Abdominal pain, headache and myalgia may also be present.

Vomiting: When *vomiting* is the major clinical feature, a virus should be suspected, e.g., rotavirus in an infant and Norwalk virus in an adult. Rotavirus causes a high percentage of diarrheal disease among infants in the United States and is more common during the winter. Norwalk virus appears to cause many cases of epidemic gastroenteritis in adults. Toxin-mediated disorders such as *Staphylococcus aureus* food poisoning also present vomiting as the major clinical feature. In staphylococcal food poisoning, the symptoms develop within one to four hours after ingesting the food containing the toxin, are usually short-lived and affect a high incidence of the population at risk. The causative organism is frequently not demonstrated in the stool. The predominance of vomiting and the short incubation period help to establish the diagnosis.

Blood: When patients pass small volume stools containing *blood* and mucus, they are said to have dysentery. Dysentery is caused by invasive bacterial pathogens that have produced inflammation of the lower gastrointestinal tract. The major agents causing dysentery are *Shigella, Campylobacter,* and occasionally *Salmonella.*

Duration: Chronic or Protracted: When diarrhea persists more than two weeks, a particular set of causes should be suspected. *Giardia lamblia* can be implicated in about a third of such patients. This is in sharp contrast to the situation with acute diarrhea where *Giardia lamblia* is the causative agent in less than 4% of patients. Because of small intestinal stasis or inhibition of motility in certain cases of diarrhea, colonic flora may overgrow in the small intestinal lumen, interfering with absorption of dietary materials. This situation leads to subacute or persistent diarrhea.

A number of individuals with more protracted diarrhea suffer from lactase deficiency induced by small intestinal infection. The disaccharidase are vulnerable because of their location on or within the microvilli of intestinal epithelial cells. Characteristically, disaccharidase deficiency may be caused by rotavirus, Norwalk virus, toxigenic *E. coli* or *Giardia.* Occasionally the bacterial pathogens such as *E. coli, Shigella, Salmonella* or *Campylobacter* can produce protracted diarrhea.

Male Homosexual

The male homosexual presents a special host for organisms causing diarrhea. Proctosigmoidoscopy is the most important screening test for these patients. The likely etiology of their illness will be determined by the level of colonic mucosal involvement as determined by endoscopy. When involvement is confined to the distal 15 cm (proctitis), a select number of organisms, generally transmitted by direct rectal inoculation, can be expected, i.e., *N. gonorrhoeae*, *H. simplex*, *C. trachomatis* (non-LGV serovats) and *T. pallidum*.

When involvement of the colonic mucosa extends beyond 15 cm, proctocolitis is diagnosed and the expected causes of colitis, i.e., *C. jejuni*, *C. fetus*, *Shigella*, *C. trachomatis* (LGV type) or *C. difficile*, should be considered. When there is no distal colonic involvement, any infectious agent can be responsible. In one study, *G. lamblia* was the most important single cause of diarrhea in this group of patients. Often, the male homosexual with diarrhea is infected with multiple agents which complicate the establishment of specific etiology. *Cryptosporidia* is an important acid-fast coccidial parasite in patients with human immunodeficiency virus infection. The workup of gay males with diarrhea is expensive and is in part guided by the results of preliminary microbiologic studies and the response to any initial empiric therapy.

Laboratory Procedures

The initial screening test for most patients with moderate to severe diarrhea is the fecal leukocyte test.[2] A methylene blue stain, used in the hematology laboratory for reticulocyte staining, can be used to stain the white cells in either a wet-mount preparation using a cover slip or by heat fixing the stool specimen and examining the slide with a dry preparation under oil. If many fecal leukocytes are present, the patient has diffuse colonic inflammation, the most common causes of which are *Shigella*, *Salmonella* and *Campylobacter*. A variety of other infectious agents or disorders may, however, be associated with diffuse inflammation of the colon. These include *Yersinia*, *Vibrio*, *Aeromonas* and inflammatory bowel disease. The conventional invasive pathogens such as *Shigella* and *Salmonella* may occasionally cause localized inflammation or involve the small intestine, in which case the stool will not show leukocytes primarily because of dilution in the large volume of colonic material.

Bacteriologic Culture

Since most stool cultures are negative when patients with diarrhea are screened to bacterial pathogens, this laboratory test should be restricted for patients likely to have a positive culture. The criteria currently recommended to select patients with diarrhea for stool cultures include: high fever (temperature greater than 101° F; severe illness requiring hospitalization; protracted diarrhea lasting more than two weeks; and the presence of leukocytes in fecal smears.

Parasitic Exam

The incidence of parasitic infection is even lower than that of bacterial infection. Therefore, selection criteria for a parasitic examination are even more restrictive. Currently we recommend parasitic exam for the following types of patients: those ill longer than two weeks; homosexual males; day care center attendees; and travelers to mountainous areas of North America or the Soviet Union.

THERAPY

Empiric Therapy

Symptomatic: Since most patients with mild to moderate acute diarrhea do not meet the criteria for stool culture or parasitic examination, it is wise to offer empiric therapy for this group. The most important therapy for these patients is fluid and electrolyte replacement. Providing dehydration is not present, the exact composition of the electrolyte solution is not very important. Patients should be encouraged to eat saltine crackers and soft drinks, such as Gatorade[R], Pedialyte[R] or other readily available solutions.

Symptomatic therapy is acceptable for moderately severe illness (approximately four unformed stools per day), where associated symptoms are not distressing. We currently use either bismuth subsalicylate Pepto-Bismol[R] in a dose of 30 ml every 30 minutes for a total of eight doses (one 8-ounce bottle in three and one half hours) or loperamide (Imodium[R]) in an initial dose of 4 mg followed by 2 mg after each unformed stool, not to exceed 16 mg per day.[3,4] These drugs may be given for a two day period. Bismuth subsalicylate usually provides a degree of symptomatic relief, with reduction in the frequency of stools and some alleviation of abdominal cramps. Loperamide also relieves cramps but has not been demonstrated to reduce the volume of fluid loss from the intestine.

Antimicrobial agents: Antimicrobial drugs are reserved for those patients with high fever, dysentery and striking illness with many fecal leukocytes, as well as for travelers with acute diarrhea. Drugs currently recommended for adults include quinolones, such as ciprofloxacin,[5,6] and norfloxacin[7] or alternatively, trimethoprim/sulfamethoxazole.[8,9]

Ciprofloxacin or norfloxacin provides excellent intestinal antibacterial concentrations, and in most instances, an infecting pathogen is rapidly eliminated from the feces. In a study of bacterial diarrhea, 38 patients were selected at random to receive ciprofloxacin (500 mg bid), and another 38 were given placebo. Diarrhea was shortened from 2.9 days to 1.5 in the placebo and active drug groups, respectively ($p<0.001$). In the two groups the number of patients with positive stool cultures one week after start of therapy were 23/36 and 2/38 in the two groups ($p<0.001$).

Organism-Specific Antimicrobial Therapy

When a specific pathogen has been identified, therapy should be given accordingly. Current recommendations for specific therapy are given in Table I.

Shigella: Shigella strains are usually resistant to ampicillin, sulfonamides, and tetracycline; and resistance to trimethoprim/sulfamethoxazole has already been observed in South America, Africa, Southeast Asia and Korea, a pattern which may well become even more widespread geographically. If the illness is acquired during travel to these regions, ciprofloxacin or norfloxacin should be prescribed, although trimethoprim/sulfamethoxazole remains a viable option at present for disease acquired in the United States and many other areas. For a child with shigellosis, trimethoprim/sulfamethoxazole can be given, while alternate drugs include nalidixic acid or furazolidone. (See Table I for dose and duration.)

Salmonella: If the patient has laboratory-confirmed *Salmonella* gastroenteritis, we generally do not give antimicrobial agents. However, ciprofloxacin has excellent activity against *Salmonella* and has been demonstrated in a recent clinical study to be effective in treating adults with salmonellosis[6] and to significantly shorten the duration of symptoms. Among 21 placebo-treated patients, the mean duration of diarrhea was 3.4 days as compared with only 1.9 days ($p<0.01$) in 16 ciprofloxacin-treated patients. This may be a worthwhile approach in selected patients with severe clinical disease. Diarrhea associated with other agents such as *Aeromonas* or *Plesiomonas* should be treated as *Shigella*.

Campylobacter: Campylobacter infection does not respond to conventional therapy for *Shigella*. A quinolone such as ciprofloxacin or norfloxacin should be given to adults, while erythromycin may be administered to children. It has been generally assumed that erythromycin is the most useful drug in human campylobacterosis. However, little information currently exists to indicate that the drug significantly shortens the duration of the clinical disease. On the other hand, *C. jejuni is* highly susceptible to quinolones *in vitro*. Pichler and colleagues,[6] demonstrated the beneficial effect of ciprofloxacin in the treatment of campylobacterosis. In 19 culture-proven cases the duration of diarrhea after ciprofloxacin treatment was begun was 1.1 days as compared to 2.2 days for placebo-treated patients ($p<0.01$). Furthermore, Goodman and colleagues,[10] using a marmoset model of *Campylobacter*-induced diarrhea, have shown that ciprofloxacin was superior to erythromycin.

Other organisms: Quinacrine is the drug of choice for laboratory-confirmed giardiasis. However, when treating a presumptive *Giardia* infection empirically, metronidazole is preferred because it is also effective against other protozoal pathogens and is probably effective in treating a bacterial overgrowth syndrome.

Entamoeba histolytica: A drug which is effective against the trophozoic form of the *E. histolytica* infection, such as metronidazole, is generally combined with a drug active against the cyst, such as diiodohydroxyquin. We generally withhold therapy for patients with cryptosporidiosis, since effective drugs are not yet available.

Traveler's diarrhea: Traveler's diarrhea (diarrhea occurring in those traveling from industrial regions to a developing tropical country) is usually caused by a bacterial agent.[1] Therefore, antimicrobial agents play an important role in prophylaxis and treatment. The current recommended treatment is trimethoprim/sulfamethoxazole.[9] We have, however, conducted a trial comparing ciprofloxacin with trimethoprim/sulfamethoxazole in 191 adult students from the United States who had acquired traveler's diarrhea in Mexico.[11] This comparative double-blind placebo-controlled trial demonstrated that both active regimens were superior to placebo and equal to each other in efficacy. The duration of diarrhea unassociated with an identifiable pathogen was also reduced by the active regimens, suggesting that unidentified bacterial pathogens may be in part responsible for this entity. Ciprofloxacin is especially suited to the treatment of acute bacterial diarrhea where trimethoprim/sulfamethoxazole resistant-strains are prevalent and where *Campylobacter* strains are common.

Diverticulitis: Patients with diverticulitis generally present with acute abdominal pain. Since the involvement often is found in the distal colon, the abdominal pain and tenderness may be over the left lower quadrant simulating "left-sided" appendicitis. Patients may have fever or a palpable mass. They often show leukocytosis and may pass blood in their stools. The therapy of diverticulitis includes drugs which have activity against both aerobic and anaerobic intestinal flora. We currently recommend the use of trimethoprim/sulfamethoxazole plus metronidazole for treatment of these patients. An alternative is doxycycline. Surgery is indicated when a patient perforates a diverticulum, a fistula is detected, or a left lower quadrant abscess is present. Surgery may be performed electively in patients who have had recurring bouts of diverticulitis. Such surgery includes drainage of any purulent material and, with extensive diverticulosis, resection of the affected area of bowel.

FUTURE CONSIDERATIONS

The recent FDA approval of ciprofloxacin and norfloxacin is important because the fluoroquinolones represent the class of drugs with the greatest future potential for the prevention and treatment of bacterial enteric infection.[12] These products are well absorbed orally and have long enough elimination half-lives to obviate the need for frequent dosing.[13] Also advantageous is the lack of plasmid-mediated resistance and the inability of bacteria to transfer resistance to other organisms.[14] Oral treatment of even serious enteric infections is frequently possible with quinolones, resulting in considerable cost savings during hospitalization and earlier discharge to home care. Quinolones also have a favorable side effect profile. Their spectrum of activity should lead to increasing usage in the treatment of a wide variety of bacterial diarrheas including those caused by *Shigella, Campylobacter,* possibly *Salmonella* and empirically in severe febrile diarrhea in which it is inappropriate to pursue the specific cause.

TABLE I. Antimicrobial agents in the therapy of infectious diarrhea

Indication	Adults	Children
Shigellosis	Trimethoprim (TMP)/ Sulfamethoxazole (SMX) 160 mg TMP/800 mg SMX bid for 3-5 days or Ciprofloxacin 500 mg or Norfloxacin 400 mg bid for 3-5 days	10 mg TMP/50 mg SMX/kg/day in two daily divided doses

TABLE I. Continued

Indication	Adults	Children
Shigellosis		Nalidixic acid 55 mg/kg/day in four daily divided doses for 5 days Furazolidone 5-7 mg/kg/day in four daily divided doses for 5 days
Salmonellosis (nontyphoid gastroenteritis)	None or Ciprofloxacin 500 mg or Norfloxacin 400 mg bid for 5 days	None
Campylobacterosis	Ciprofloxacin 500 mg or Norfloxacin 400 mg bid for 5 days	Erythromycin 50 mg/kg/day in four equal doses for 5 days
Traveler's Diarrhea	Same as Shigellosis	Same as Shigellosis
Giardiasis	Quinacrine 100 mg tid or Metronidazole 250 mg tid	Quinacrine 7 mg/kg/day, orally three times a day for 7-10 days Metronidazole 20 mg/kg/day, four times a day for 10 days
Amebiasis	Metronidazole 750 mg tid for 5 days plus Diiodohydroxyquin 650 mg orally tid for 21 days	Metronidazole 50 mg/kg/day for 5 days plus Diiodohydroxyquin 40 mg/kg/day in three doses for 21 days

Acute Diarrhea

Most common clinical presentation of enteric infection
Increase in stool number, decrease in form >200 gm/day

Epidemiologic Associations

Presence of associated cases
Travel
Prior antimicrobial therapy
Day care center exposure
Homosexual male

Clinical Features

Fever	- Invasive pathogens
Vomiting	- Viruses, toxin-mediated
Dysentery	- Colonic inflammation
Persistent or subacute illness	- *Giardia*, overgrowth, lactase deficiency, bacterial pathogens

Male Homosexual

Proctitis	- *N. gonorrhoeae, H. simplex C. trachomatis, T. pallidum*
Proctocolitis	- *C. jejuni, C. fetus, Shigella, C. trachomatis, C. difficile*
Enteritis	*Giardia*, etc.

Laboratory Procedures

Fecal leukocyte test Indicates diffuse colonic inflammation

TABLE I. Continued

Laboratory Procedures

Bacteriologic culture	High fever, severe illness, protracted illness, fecal leukocytes

Laboratory Procedures

Parasite exam	Chronicity, homosexual male, day care center exposure, travel to mountainous areas of Soviet Union

Empiric Therapy

Fluids/electrolytes	
Symptomatic therapy	Bismuth subsalicylate
	Loperamide

Antimicrobial therapy with high fever, dysentery, fecal leukocytes, in travelers TMP/SMX vs quinolone (adults)

Laboratory Confirmed Illness

Shigella	TMP/SMX	
Salmonella	None, consider quinolone (adults)	
Aeromonas, Plesiomonas		TMP/SMX, or quinolone (adults)
	Erythromycin (children)	
Giardia	Quinacrine	
E. histolytica	Metronidazole + Diiodohydroxyquin	
Cryptosporidium	None	

Diverticulitis

Abdominal pain, tenderness ("left-sided appendicitis")
Other findings: fever, leukocytosis, palpable mass, bleeding

Therapy Diverticulosis

Aerobic	TMP/SMX
Anaerobic	Metronidazole
Alternative	Doxycycline
Surgery	for perforation, fistula formation or abscess or electively for recurrent attacks.

REFERENCES

1. DuPont HL, Pickering LK. In: DuPont HL, Pickering LK, eds. Infections of the gastrointestinal tract: microbiology, pathophysiology, and clinical features. New York: Plenum Publishing Co., 1980.
2. Harris JC, DuPont HL, Hornick RB. Fecal leukocytes in diarrheal illness. Ann Intern Med 1972;76:697-703.
3. DuPont HL, Sullivan P, Pickering LK, et al. Symptomatic treatment of diarrhea with bismuth subsalicylate among students attending a Mexican university. Gastroenterol 1977; 73:715-8.
4. DuPont HL. Nonfluid therapy and selected chemoprophylaxis of acute diarrhea. Am J Med 1985;78:Suppl 6B:81-90.
5. DuPont HL, Ericsson CD, Robinson A, et al. Current problems in antimicrobial therapy for bacterial enteric infection. Am J Med 1987;82:Suppl 4A:324-8.
6. Pichler HET, Piridl G, Stickler K, et al. Clinical efficacy of ciprofloxacin compared with placebo in bacterial diarrhea. Am J Med 1987;82:Suppl 4A:329-32.
7. DuPont HL, Corrado ML, Sabbaj J. The use of norfloxacin in the treatment of acute diarrheal disease. Am J Med 1987; 82:Suppl 6B:79-83.
8. Nelson JD, Kusmiesz H, Jackson LH, et al. Trimethoprim/sulfamethoxazole therapy for shigellosis. JAMA 1976;235:1239-43.

9. DuPont HL, Reves RR, Galindo E, et al. Treatment of travelers dealing with trimethoprim/sulfamethoxazole and with trimethoprim alone. N Engl J Med 1982;307:841-4.
10. Goodman LJ, Kaplan RL, Petrak RM, et al. Effects of erythromycin and ciprofloxacin on chronic excretion of *Campylobacter* species. Antimicrob Agents Chemother 1986;29:185-7.
11. Ericsson CD, Johnson PC, DuPont HL, et al. Ciprofloxacin or trimethoprim - sulfamethoxazole as initial therapy for travelers' diarrhea. Ann Intern Med 1987;106:216-20.
12. DuPont HL. Quinolone antimicrobial agents in the management of bacterial enteric infections. In: Wolfson JS, Hooper DC, eds. Quinolone antimicrobial agents. Washington, DC: Am Soc Microbiol 1989:8:167-176.
13. Drusano GL. Pharmacokinetics of the quinolone antimicrobial agents. In: Wolfson JS, Hooper DC, eds. Quinolone antimicrobial agents. Washington, DC: Am Soc Microbiol 1989:4:71-105.
14. Burman LG. Apparent absence of transferable resistance to nalidixic acid in pathogenic gram negative bacteria. J Antimicrob Chemother 1977;3:509-1.

CHAPTER 11

Ambulatory Treatment of Patients Infected with Human Immunodeficiency Virus (HIV)

Laurence M. Cortez, M.D.
New Orleans, Louisiana

INTRODUCTION

There is no question as to the desirability of treating Human Immunodeficiency Virus (HIV) infected patients in the outpatient setting rather than in the hospital, regardless of the state of disease. The patients usually prefer avoidance of the hospital setting and fare much better psychologically when treated on an outpatient basis. Cost is a consideration when choosing the site of care. The average cost of medical care for Acquired Immune Deficiency Syndrome (AIDS) patients has dropped at least 50% since the onset of the epidemic, while the life expectancy has lengthened. These benefits are due to better success in preventing and treating opportunistic infections, as well as to an improved network of support groups, home health services and hospices. Still, an estimated $65 billion annually will be needed to care for this cohort of patients.[1] Preventative medicine and outpatient care are critical aspects of care for HIV infected patients.

PNEUMOCYSTIS CARINII

Pneumocystis carinii pneumonia (PCP) has been the most common life-threatening opportunistic infection occurring in AIDS patients. PCP accounts for 65% of the initial infections seen in AIDS patients[2] and can be found in 20%[1] of patients with already established diagnosis of AIDS by other criteria. Based on projections of 270,000 cases of AIDS in the United States by 1991[3] a cumulative total of at least 200,000 cases of PCP can be expected. Also, recurrences of PCP are not infrequent due to persistence of the organism. In fact, even when clinical resolution has occurred, cysts and trophozoites of PCP have been demonstrated in the lungs of the involved individuals. At the onset of the AIDS epidemic, the survival rate of the first episode of PCP was 75%-80%, with a survival rate of 25%-35% following the second bout. Now, the incidence of survival is 90% for a first bout of PCP, 80% for a second bout, and there are survivors of even third and fourth episodes.

Therefore, because of the high incidence of AIDS patients who contract PCP, and because of the great likelihood for repeated bouts, it is warranted to try to prevent initial episodes, as well as recurrences, of PCP. Drugs used for therapy would be likely candidates for use in prevention. Also, for financial and other practical reasons, prophylaxis should be administered in the outpatient setting.

FIGURE 1. Agents used for prevention of PCP in HIV patients

1. Trimethoprim/sulfamethoxazole (TMP/SMX)
2. Sulfadoxine-pyrimethamine (Fansidar[R])
3. Dapsone
4. Pentamidine (IM or IV)
5. Pentamidine (Aerosolized)

Both TMP/SMX and pentamidine have 80% efficacy rates as therapy for the first episodes of PCP.[4] Effectiveness of TMP/SMX in the prevention of PCP has been demonstrated in AIDS patients[6] and in children with acute lymphocytic leukemia.[5] However, TMP/SMX and parenteral pentamidine are not well tolerated by AIDS patients. Side effects necessitating discontinuation of the drug occur in at least 50% of patients.[4,6,7,8] AIDS patients treated successfully for PCP with TMP/SMX might tolerate TMP/SMX prophylactically.

Conflicting opinions exist on the efficacy of sulfadoxine-pyrimethamine for PCP in AIDS patients. In addition, there have been recent reports of fatal reactions with sulfadoxine-pyrimethamine.[3] This drug might, however, offer the advantage of possible prevention of toxoplasmosis activation, an ever increasing problem, but at present there have been no controlled studies.

Controlled studies of dapsone have not as yet been reported, and it is quite unlikely that such studies will be initiated since aerosolized pentamidine is now available to physicians and most are prescribing it without awaiting additional data. In fact, any similar product developed will more than likely be required to be studied in comparison to aerosolized pentamidine. However, the efficacy for prophylaxis of aerosolized pentamidine appears to be such that many patients would most likely not consent to a comparison drug, and one must question the ethicality of administering a comparison drug under such desperate circumstances.

The ideal agent for treatment of any infectious disease is one that eliminates the organism selectively at the site of infection without toxicity. Since *Pneumocystis carinii* are located within the alveolar spaces, one might expect pentamidine administered by inhalation to be effective, site specific, and less toxic systemically.

Armstrong and colleagues using bioassay techniques on autopsy specimens of patients who had received parenteral pentamidine, found that drug levels in the liver, kidneys, adrenals and spleen were higher than in the lungs.[9] Disease caused by PCP is rare outside of the lung.[10] Therapeutic levels of pentamidine in rat lungs after inhalation were demonstrated by Waldeman in 1973.[11] Montgomery and colleagues have demonstrated high levels of pentamidine in human bronchiolar lavage sediment after IV doses.[12] Bernard and Armstrong have demonstrated the efficacy of inhaled pentamidine in preventing and treating PCP in rats.[13]

Armstrong also noted that levels of 20 ug/gm-30 ug/gm of lung tissue were achieved only after four to five days of administering parenteral pentamidine. This may explain why it frequently takes several days to see clinical improvement. High levels of the drug were maintained for up to two weeks after the last dose. These pharmacologic factors suggest that once a patient passes the first four to five days of therapy, daily treatment with parenteral pentamidine may not be necessary. While the validity of this approach has yet to be evaluated, it may be possible that pentamidine can be administered every several days, or concomitant aerosolized pentamidine can be administered and then used to complete therapy.

Table I presents a partial listing of abstracts of papers suggesting efficacy of aerosolized pentamidine in the prophylaxis of PCP that were presented at the 1988 annual meeting of the American Thoracic Society[14] and at the June, 1988 IV International Conference on AIDS in Stockholm.[15] It should be noted that dose, particle size, frequency of administration, importance of reservoirs, external filters, flow rates, position of the patient, etc., are physical factors that need to be determined in order to offer the best chance of success. These factors may differ from patient to patient, depending on presence or absence of obstruction or restriction or other pulmonary factors.

The particle size needs to be between one and two micra for alveolar deposition.[16] The nebulizer must maximize deposition in the alveoli while minimizing deposition in the large airways, since the sulfur moiety in pentamidine isethionate is an airways irritant.[17] If the particles are too large, they never reach the invasive area; if they are too small, they escape in a gaseous phase.

It should be noted that the only measure of occurrence over time can be seen in patients with previous episodes of PCP. In most of these studies, percentages are not expressed in terms of rates of recurrence. Therefore, it is difficult to reliably compare the results of these reports.

TABLE I. Summary of studies using aerosolized pentamidine (from references 14 and 15)

Author(s)	# Pts	Dose	Interval	Average Duration	Prior PCP	% PCP
Van Gundy	33	2 mg/kg	2 wks	18 wks	33	7
Fallat	188	30 mg	2 wks	?	159	9.6
Van Gundy	56	60 mg	2 wks	70 days	?	24
Van Gundy	56	150 mg	2 wks	147 days	?	6
Smith	12	300 mg	2 wks	16 wks	12	0
Conte	93	300 mg	4 wks	3.1 mos (mean)	48	3.2
Leoung/ Montgomery	433	30 mg 150 mg 300 mg	2 wks 2 wks 4 wks	106 days (mean)	250	2.8
Gabin	150	60 mg	1 wk X 4 then 2 wks	?	?	1 in 8 mos
Bernard/ Armstrong	162	60 mg	1 wk X 4 then 2 wks	7.1 mos (mean)	143	2.5
Van Gundy	29	2 mg/kg	2 wks	26 wks	29	13.7
Girard	92	4 mg/kg	2 wks X 2 then 4 wks	12.1 wks (mean)	75	3.3

NB: Historical control recurrence rate = 35% in 180 days

In Van Gundy's first abstract, the particle size was not given (see Table I.). In the second and third, which are, in fact, one study the first 60 patients who had a high recurrence rate of 24%, received a 60 mg dose with a nebulizer that delivered particle sizes of 10 to 20 micra. Gabin used the Respirgard II nebulizer, which is the one presently being used by many investigators.[14,15]

It should be noted that historically, 35% of patients will have a recurrence within 180 days following their first episode of PCP.

Conte commented that the maximum course was 5.2 months and that the three relapses seen, compared to ten on the basis of historical controls, were delayed by at least five months in patients with one preceding episode of PCP.[14,15] Leoung and Montgomery noted that the number of relapses in 152 historical controls with a single previous episode of PCP was 37, as compared to six relapses in 152 patients on aerosolized pentamidine.[14,15]

Bernard and Armstrong expressed their results as the rate of PCP/100 patient months. In this study, the number of recurrences of patients using aerosolized pentamidine was 0.35/100 patient months as compared to 3.4/100 patient months in an earlier trial using a less efficient nebulizer. When no prophylaxis was given after a first episode of PCP, the rate of recurrence was 4.6/100 patient months.[14,15]

For patients using aerosolized pentamidine, toxicity has been noted in about 5% to 7% of cases and consists primarily of bronchospasm, which can usually be prevented with slower administration. There have been no adverse effects noted on pulmonary function. Complaints of bad taste are common.

These studies suggest that aerosolized pentamidine can be of great value in prevention of PCP and can be considered relatively safe. It is very difficult to do blind, random, or comparative trials with aerosolized pentamidine, just as it is for many drugs tested for AIDS patients, due to the uniform rapidity of morbidity and mortality associated with this infection. However, with the increasing large number of patients being treated, it should soon be possible for some standardization of therapy to be achieved, perhaps enabling meaningful comparative trials of this mode of therapy to be performed. Importantly, if, in a given geographic location, it is difficult for a patient to come to the physician's office for inhalations, this can be accomplished at home.

Therefore, in light of these studies, it seems appropriate to give pentamidine inhalations to all HIV infected patients. The optimum dose and frequency have yet to be determined. At our institution, we are currently administering 300 mg every four weeks. Of note, in June 1989, the FDA approved prophylaxis with aerosolized pentamdine in a dose of 300 mg every four weeks for patients with prior episodes of PCP or CD_4 counts $< 200/mm^3$.

CRYPTOCOCCUS NEOFORMANS

Cryptococcosis is the fourth most common opportunistic infection seen in AIDS patients, occurring in 6% to 13.3% of cases.[17,18] The infection is disseminated in 50%, but clinical symptomatology is most often reflected in the central nervous system, with lung involvement being second. Cryptococcus is second only to *Toxoplasma gondii as* an opportunistic infection of the CNS of AIDS patients.

Overall mortality of cryptococcosis in AIDS patients is 60%.[19] Relapse occurs in 50% to 90% of those patients who initially respond to therapy and is associated with a 100% mortality.[19,20] The overall survival is only five months.[21] Usually, infected patients have an additional opportunistic infection and/or malignancy.

Cryptococcus may be very indolent and symptomatology may be vague, with infrequent focal neurologic signs. Most often, patients present only with headache, anorexia, nausea, fever, or a change in sensorium. In any HIV positive patient, even these subtle symptoms should initiate consideration of central nervous system HIV, toxoplasmosis, cryptococcosis, cytomegalovirus, lymphoma, or other neoplastic disease.

Diagnosis is based on clinical suspicion leading to appropriate stains and cultures of blood, spinal fluid, and tissue specimens, as well as to latex agglutination for cryptococcal antigen in the blood, spinal fluid and urine. The presence of cryptococcal antigen means infection. A prozone phenomenon may occur in patients with high titers resulting in a false negative test. If one's index of suspicion is high and the cryptococcal antigen is negative, further dilutions should be done on the samples and repeat determinations performed.

Treatment of *Cryptococcus* with Amphotericin

Amphotericin B 0.5 mg/kg/day to 1.0 mg/kg/day until one to two grams is given has been the mainstay of therapy. The addition of 5-flucytosin (5-FC) has not been beneficial,[20] and its toxicities appear to be exaggerated in AIDS patients. Serum antigen titers may remain stable, increase or decrease without clinical correlation. CSF titers usually fall with effective therapy. Without therapy, titers higher than 1:8 are associated with relapse,[18,22] and in one study, CSF antigen titers greater than 1:1000 were associated with 100% mortality.[20]

The standard induction dose is one to two grams of Amphotericin B, followed by maintenance therapy three times per week. Administration is IV but can be accomplished in the home or office. The limiting factor to home administration is toxicity, both immediate (fever, shaking chills, headache, nausea, etc.) and long term (nephrotoxicity, hepatotoxicity, bone marrow toxicity, etc.). Prophylactic measures for decreasing immediate reaction include:

1. Benadryl[R]
2. Demerol[R]
3. Acetaminophin
4. NSAIDS
5. Hydrocortisone PO4

All may be used on *outpatients.*

Immediate toxicity can usually be prevented by premedication with indomethacin 50 mg orally and diphenhydramine 50 mg orally one hour prior to onset or IV plus meperidine 50 mg to 75 mg IV for the development of any symptoms.

Treatment of *Cryptococcus*
Fluconazole

Fluconazole is a new triazole antifungal agent, developed by Pfizer, which has a broad antifungal spectrum, a greater than 90% absorption after an oral dose, a long half-life with little metabolism (60% to 80% excreted unchanged in the urine), and saliva, sputum, blister fluid, peritoneal fluid and vaginal tissue levels equal to levels achieved in plasma. CSF levels are 50% to 90% of plasma levels. Minor GI upsets occur in about 10% of patients; reversible changes in liver function tests occur in under 5% of patients.

Preliminary data from patients participating in the National Institute of Allergy and Infectious Disease Mycosis Study Group suggest efficacy of fluconazole

(200/mg orally daily) in the treatment of cryptococcal meningitis in AIDS patients. This finding is supported by two case reports,[23,24] and our experience with four patients is also encouraging. Fluconazole is currently available for compassionate use from Dr. Anthony K. Kuirsch of Pfizer Central Research, Groton, Connecticut (203) 441-4811.

TABLE II. Fluconazole characteristics

Mechanism of action: inhibits ergosterol synthesis
Absorption: 90+%
T 1/2 = 25-30 hours
Excretion = 60-80% unchanged in urine
Protein binding = 11%
Water soluble
Concentrations: saliva, sputum, blister fluid,
peritoneal fluid = plasma level
urine, skin = 10 x plasma level
CSF = 50 - 90% plasma level

FIGURE 2. Case history of a patient with *Cryptococcus* treated with Fluconazole

42 year old homosexual male. Positive HIV aby 5/85.
asymptomatic till:
4/87 headache & low grade fever
T-helper count - 7
CT Scan = negative
CSF = 4 WBC's (79% L, 8% S, 13% M)
6 RBC's, Glu = 50, Pro = 40
India Ink = positive
Culture = positive
Cryptococcal antigen:
Serum = 1 : 1,024
CSF = 1 : 128
Amphotericin B 25 mg/d X 14 days.
A Hickman catheter was placed and outpatient therapy continued with amphotericin B 50 mg MWF.
5/87 TB/DB = 1.6/1.0; SGOT = 530, SGPT = 242
Alk phos = 1,241
6/87 Mild headache and intermittent fever persisted.
T helper = 24
Cryptococcal antigen
Serum = **NEGATIVE**. Prozone
phenomenon; diluted =
1 : 32,768
CSF = 1 : 256
Cholestatic jaundice:
TB/DB = 3/2.3 Alk phos = 2,050
SGOT = 66, SGPT = 58
Renal Tubular Acidosis:
HCO3 - 19
Hgb = 7.5, WBC = 2,000
Amphotericin B decreased to 30 mg M&Th
7/87 Cryptococcol antigen:
Serum = 1: 32,768

FIGURE 2. Continued

	CSF = 1: 256
	SGOT - 100, SGPT = 100
	Alk phos = 398
8/87	SGOT = 60, SGPT = 60
	Alk phos = 250
	Amphotericin B increased to 30 mg M-F
9/87	Progressive deteriorization
	Cryptococcal antigen:
	Serum = 1: 32, 768
	SCF = 1:16, 384
	CSF: 42 WBC's (100%) Glucose = 7,
	Protein = 124
	Culture = heavy growth
	AZT started, discontinued after 2 weeks
10/87	Demented, incontinent
	admitted for terminal care
	CSF antigen = 1: 8, 142
10/2/87	Fluconazole 400 mg/day p.o. begun
10/15/87	Alert, oriented, walking
	Full return to baseline mental status
10/30/87	CSF fluconazole = plasma fluconazole
	CSF: 16 WBC's (96% L, 4% M), Glucose = 8
	Protein = 290
	Culture = **NEGATIVE**
11/87	CSF: 2 WBC's
	Culture = negative
	Crypotococcal antigen:
	Serum = 1: 4, 096
	CSF = 1: 8, 192
1/88	CSF culture = negative
3/88	CSF culture = negative
	Cryptococcal antigen:
	Serum = 1: 32, 768
	CSF = 1: 8, 192
6/88	Continued to do well neurologically
	Intraoral lymphoma noted
	Resolved with radiation treatment
7/88	Acute intestinal obstruction secondary to bowel lymphoma.
	Ventilator dependent post op.
	Died of sepsis and disseminated lymphoma
	Autopsy: Cultures:
	No fungi recovered from CSF or brain
	Path:
	Brain - full of cryptococci
	Parenchymal cysts full of cryptococci
	Meninges - cloudy and thickened
	Lymphoma in GI tract and mouth

This case demonstrated the inaccuracy of cryptococcal antigen results in following the course of the illness. An inability to clear the antigen from the CSF may account for this situation. This case also clearly demonstrates the inability of therapy to "cure" opportunistic infections in the face of ongoing immunosuppression. However, fluconazole obviously suppressed progression of infection sufficiently to prolong life and to enhance the quality of the young man's remaining days.

OTHER FUNGI

Amphotericin B remains the treatment of choice for other systemic fungi, such as histoplasmosis and coccidioidomycosis. Patients need to be maintained for life on antifungal therapy, which can be accomplished with oral ketoconazole and, quite likely, with fluconazole, itraconazole, or other triazoles currently under development.

Chronic or recurrent *Candida* can be suppressed with a variety of nystatin or clotrimazole preparations administered topically. When these do not suffice, ketoconazole 200 mg to 400 mg per day is usually effective.

HERPES VIRUSES

Most adults with AIDS have already been infected with Herpes Simplex Virus (HSV) types I and II. Reactivation of latent infection and recurrent disease are common, especially in homosexual males who have a high incidence of HSV antibodies indicating previous infection.[25]

Ulcerative lesions persisting for greater than one month without evidence of other cause of immune suppression or positive HIV serology fulfill the criteria for the diagnosis of AIDS. Oral, orolabial, genital, anorectal, and esophageal involvement all commonly occur in AIDS patients. Encephalitis does occur, but infrequently.

Standard initial therapy for HSV in AIDS patients is acyclovir. Acyclovir-resistant HSV does occur and can be treated with vidarabine 15 mg/kg/day for at least ten days.[26]

TABLE III. Therapy of HSV in AIDS

Clinical Category	Regimen
Severe mucocutaneous	Acyclovir: 15 mg/kg/day IV
Mild mucocutaneous	Acyclovir: 200 mg po 5X/day
Disseminated	Acyclovir: 30 mg/kg/day IV
Recurrent mucocutaneous	Acyclovir: 200-400 mg po tid-qid
Significant acyclovir resistant infection	Vidarabine: 15 mg/kg/day IV

Varicella-Zoster Virus

Most adults have been previously exposed to varicella-zoster virus (VZ), but primary infection can occur in AIDS patients and may be life-threatening.

Recurrent VZ infection, shingles or localized zoster, may be treated orally. Clinical judgment dictates whether patients need hospitalization for treatment of initial infections since patients with initial infections are at high risk for dissemintion associated with significant mortality. Intravenous therapy or observation in a hospital setting may be warranted for such patients. Table IV should provide therapeutic regimen of VZ. Therapy is continued until clusters are gone.

TABLE IV. Therapy of VZV in AIDS

Clinical Category	Regimen
Primary Varicella or Zoster (shingles, recurrent localized)	Acyclovir: 30 mg/kg/day IV or 600-800 mg po 5X/day
Disseminated (recurrent)	Acyclovir: 30 mg/kg/day IV or 600-800 mg po 5X/day

Cytomegalovirus

Cytomegalovirus (CMV) is the most common opportunistic viral cause of life-threatening infection in AIDS cases. Nearly 100% of homosexual men with HIV have serological evidence of CMV. Retinitis, colitis, gastritis, esophagitis, pneumonitis, hepatitis[27] and encephalitis occur. Involvement of the spleen, kidneys, pancreas,[28] adrenals,[27] and epididymis[29] have been documented. With the exception of the eye involvement (CMV retinitis), it may be difficult to distinguish colonization from true infection. Clinical response to ganciclovir supports the diagnosis of CMV infection.

TABLE V. Ganciclovir therapy for CMV in AIDS

Induction: 2.5 mg/kg IV q8h or 5 mg/kg IV q12h X 10-14 days

Maintenance: 5-7.5 mg/kg IV daily 5 days a week

Ganciclovir has a chemical structure similar to acyclovir. It is converted intracellularly to a DNA polymerase inhibitor. Neutropenia occurs in 25% to 50% of treated patients, and thrombocytopenia occurs in 10% of patients. Hepatotoxicity, mental status changes, rash, eosinophilia, GI upsets, and pain with or without phlebitis at the infusion site are seen less frequently. All adverse reactions appear to be rapidly reversible with discontinuation or reduction of dose.

Relapse, however, is the rule rather than the exception in CMV retinitis. And, as currently administered, it appears that ganciclovir can suppress, but not cure, CMV infections.

However, experience at our institution with ganciclovir has been gratifying and the product has recently received FDA approval for CMV retinitis. The following is the clinical course of a patient recently treated with the product.

FIGURE 3. 31 year old homosexual male noted to be HIV positive 11/86

6/87 PCP T helper = 27
Successful therapy
AZT 200 mg q 4h - good compliance

FIGURE 3. Continued

	AZT induced anemia.	Transfusion dependent. 3 units/month
1/88	Aerosolized pentamidine 120 mg q 2 wks.	
4/88	T helper = 0	
6/88	Abrupt onset nausea, vomiting, diarrhea and decreased peripheral vision OS	
	Rapid CMV urine culture positive at 24h	
	Rapid CMV blood culture positive at 24h	
	CMV colitis (histopathology)	
	Ophthalmology = CMV retinitis	
	Ganciclovir 5mg/kg q 12h IV administered for 2 wks	
	Diarrhea ceased within 24 hours.	
	Nausea ceased in 36 hours and patient requesting	
	extra meals at 48 hours	
	Vision stable at 48 hours	
	Hickman catheter placed	
	Ganciclovir 5mg/kg/day IV administered M-F	
	CBC, Platelet count, Chem 20 panel weekly	
9/88	Vision deteriorating after 7 weeks of maintenance therapy	
	T helper = 0	
	Reinduction with ganciclovir 5 mg/kg IV q12h for 2 weeks	

This man left the hospital while still on induction therapy to be supplied with premixed IV fluids containing ganciclovir for home administration via his Hickman catheter. Ganciclovir has sight-and life-saving properties for CMV infections in AIDS patients but is not curative.

As discussed earlier in this chapter in regard to pentamidine inhalations, the need to administer ganciclovir on ethical grounds will make true comparative studies or blind studies difficult, if not impossible, to perform but we can be optimistic that its development will lead to other modes of therapy down the road. An oral preparation is being developed.

In the meantime, emphasis will continue on therapies that can be administered in the outpatient setting, which is preferable to all concerned.

Necessity being the mother of invention, novel means of providing parenteral therapy in the outpatient setting will continue to be developed.

REFERENCES

1. Hopewell PC. Diagnosis of PCP. Infect Dis Clin North Am 1988;2:409-16.
2. CDC. Aids Weekly Surveillance October 12, 1987.
3. El-Sadr W, Sidhu G. Persistence of trophozoites after successful treatment of *Pneumocystis carinii* pneumonia. Ann Intern Med 1986;105:889-90.
4. Wharton JM, Coleman DL, Wofsy CM, et. al. Trimethoprim-sulfamethoxazole or pentamidine for *Pneumocystis carinii* pneumonia in the acquired immunodefiency syndrome: a prospective randomized trial. Ann Intern Med 1986;105:37-44.
5. Hughes WT, Gaston KR, et al. Successful intermittent chemoprophylaxis for *Pneumocystis carinii* pneumonitis. N Engl J Med 1987;1316:627-32.
6. Fischl MA, Dickinson GM, La Voie L. Safety and efficacy of sulfamethoxazole and trimethoprim chemoprophylaxis for *Pneumocystis carinii* pneumonia in AIDS. JAMA 1988;259:1185-9.

7. Kovacs JA, Hiemenz JW, Macher AM, et al. *Pneumocystis carinii* pneumonia: a comparison between patients with the acquired immunodeficiency syndrome and patients with other immunodeficiencies. Ann Intern Med 1984; 100:663-71.
8. Gordin FM, Simon GL, Wofsy CB, et al. Adverse reactions to trimethoprim - sulfamethoxazole in patients with the acquired immunodeficiency syndrome. Ann Intern Med 1984;100:495-9.
9. Donnelly H, Bernard EM, Rothkotter H, et al. Distribution of pentamidine in patients with AIDS. J Infect Dis 1988;157:985-9.
10. Hughes WT. Pathology. In: Hughes WT, ed. *Pneumocystis carinii* pneumonia. Boca Raton, Florida: CRC Press Inc., 1987:105-25.
11. Waldeman RH, Pearce DE, Martin RA. Pentamidine isothionate in lungs, livers and kidneys of rats after aerosol or intramuscular administration. Am Rev Respir Dis 1973;108:1004-6.
12. Montgomery AB, Debs RJ, Luce JM, et al. Selective delivery of pentamidine to the lung by aerosol. Am Rev Respir Dis 1988;137(2):477-8.
13. Bernard EM, Donnelly HJ, Huang A, et al. Successful prevention and treatment of experimental *Pneumocystis carinii* pneumonia with aerosol pentamidine. Abstracts of II International Conference on AIDS, Paris. 1986:54.
14. American Thoracic Society, 1988 Annual Meeting, Las Vegas, May 8-11, 1988 (presentations and abstracts).
15. Fourth International Conference on AIDS, Stockholm, June 12-16, 1988 (presentations and abstracts).
16. Newman SP. Aerosol deposition considerations in inhalation therapy. Chest 1985;88(Suppl):152S-160S.
17. Fine JM, Gordon T, Sheppard D. The role of pH and ionic species in sulfur dioxide and sulfite-induced bronchoconstriction. Am Rev Respir Dis 1987;136:1122-6.
18 Eng RH, Bishurg E, Smith SM, et al. Cryptococcal infections in patients with acquired immune deficiency syndrome. Am J Med 1986;81:19-23.
19. Kovacs JA, Kovacs AA, Polis M, et al. Cryptococcosis in the acquired immunodeficiency syndrome. Ann Intern Med 1985;103:533-8.
20. Zugar A, Louie E, Holzman RS, et al. Cryptococcal disease in patients with the acquired immunodeficiency syndrome. Ann Intern Med 1986;104:234-40.
21. Gal AA, Koss MN, Hawkins J, et al. The pathology of pulmonary infections in the acquired immunodeficiency syndrome. Arch Pathol Lab Med 1986;110:502-7.
22. Young LS. Management of opportunistic infection complicating the acquired immunodeficiency syndrome. Med Clin North Am 1986;70:677-92.
23. Dupont B, Drouhet E. Cryptococcal meningitis and fluconazole (letter). Ann Intern Med 1987;106:778.
24. Shelhaner JH, Ognibene FP, Macaher AM, et al. Persistence of *Pneumocystis carinii* in lung tissue of acquired immunodeficiency syndrome patients treated for pneumocystis pneumonia. Am Rev Respir Dis 1984;130:1161-5.
25. Nerurkar L, Goedert J, Wallen W, et al. Study of antiviral antibodies in sera of homosexual men. J Fed Proc 1983;42:6109.
26. Whitley RJ, Soong SJ, Dolin R, et al. Adenine arabinoside therapy of biopsy proved herpes simplex encephalitis: National Institute of Allergy and Infectious Diseases collaborated antiviral study. N Engl J Med 1977;297:289-94.
27. Reichert CM, O'Leary TJ, Levens DL, et al. Autopsy pathology in the acquired immunodeficiency syndrome. Am J Pathol 1983;12:357-82.

28. Pass HI, Potter DA, Macher AM, et al. Thoracic manifestations of the acquired immunodeficiency syndrome. J Thorac Cardiovasc Surg 1984;88:654-8.
29. Randazzo RF, Hulette CM, Cottlieb MS, et al. Cytomegalovirus epididymitis in a patient with acquired immune deficiency syndrome. J Urol 1986; 136:1095-7.